Numbers and Operations
© Mometrix Media – flashcardsecrets.com/teas
ATI TEAS Mathematics

What are integers, prime numbers, and composite numbers?

Numbers and Operations
© Mometrix Media – flashcardsecrets.com/teas
ATI TEAS Mathematics

What are even and odd numbers?

Numbers and Operations
© Mometrix Media – flashcardsecrets.com/teas
ATI TEAS Mathematics

What are decimal numbers, decimal points, and decimal places?

Numbers and Operations
© Mometrix Media – flashcardsecrets.com/teas
ATI TEAS Mathematics

What are the names of the place values of the decimal 0.123?

Numbers and Operations
© Mometrix Media – flashcardsecrets.com/teas
ATI TEAS Mathematics

Describe the decimal system and the binary system.

Numbers and Operations
© Mometrix Media – flashcardsecrets.com/teas
ATI TEAS Mathematics

What are rational, irrational, and real numbers?

Visit *mometrix.com/academy* for related videos.
Enter video codes: 461071, 280645 and 565581

Even number – any integer that can be divided by 2 without leaving a remainder. For example: 2, 4, 6, 8, and so on.

Odd number – any integer that cannot be divided evenly by 2. For example: 3, 5, 7, 9, and so on.

Integer – any positive or negative whole number, including zero. Integers do not include fractions $\left(\frac{1}{3}\right)$, decimals (0.56), or mixed numbers $\left(7\frac{3}{4}\right)$.

Prime number – any whole number greater than 1 that has only two factors, itself and 1; that is, a number that can be divided evenly only by 1 and itself.

Composite number – any whole number greater than 1 that has more than two different factors; in other words, any whole number that is not a prime number. For example: The composite number 8 has the factors of 1, 2, 4, and 8.

In the decimal 0.123, the 1 is in the first place to the right of the decimal point, indicating tenths; the 2 is in the second place, indicating hundredths; and the 3 is in the third place, indicating thousandths.

Decimal number – any number that uses a decimal point to show the part of the number that is less than one. Example: 1.234.

Decimal point – a symbol used to separate the ones place from the tenths place in decimals or dollars from cents in currency.

Decimal place – the position of a number to the right of the decimal point.

Rational numbers include all integers, decimals, and fractions. Any terminating or repeating decimal number is a rational number.

Irrational numbers cannot be written as fractions or decimals because the number of decimal places is infinite and there is no recurring pattern of digits within the number. For example, pi (π) begins with 3.141592 and continues without terminating or repeating, so pi is an irrational number.

Real numbers are the set of all rational and irrational numbers.

The **decimal**, or base 10, system is a number system that uses ten different digits (0, 1, 2, 3, 4, 5, 6, 7, 8, 9).

An example of a number system that uses something other than ten digits is the **binary**, or base 2, number system, used by computers, which uses only the numbers 0 and 1.

Numbers and Operations
© Mometrix Media – flashcardsecrets.com/teas
ATI TEAS Mathematics

Write the place value of each digit for the following number: 14,059.826

Numbers and Operations
© Mometrix Media – flashcardsecrets.com/teas
ATI TEAS Mathematics

Write each number in words: 29 | 478 | 9,435 | 98,542 | 302,876.

Numbers and Operations
© Mometrix Media – flashcardsecrets.com/teas
ATI TEAS Mathematics

Write each decimal in words: 0.06 | 0.6 | 6.0 | 0.009 | 0.113 | 0.901

Numbers and Operations
© Mometrix Media – flashcardsecrets.com/teas
ATI TEAS Mathematics

What is a fraction?

Numbers and Operations
© Mometrix Media – flashcardsecrets.com/teas
ATI TEAS Mathematics

What does a fraction represent?

Numbers and Operations
© Mometrix Media – flashcardsecrets.com/teas
ATI TEAS Mathematics

What do the numerator and the denominator of a fraction represent?

29: twenty-nine

478: four hundred seventy-eight

9,435: nine thousand four hundred thirty-five

98,542: ninety-eight thousand five hundred forty-two

302876: three hundred two thousand eight hundred seventy-six

1: ten thousands
4: thousands
0: hundreds
5: tens
9: ones
8: tenths
2: hundredths
6: thousandths

A **fraction** is a number that is expressed as one integer written above another integer, with a dividing line between them $\left(\frac{x}{y}\right)$.

0.06: six hundredths
0.6: six tenths
6.0: six

0.009: nine thousandths;
0.113: one hundred thirteen thousandths;
0.901: nine hundred and one thousandths

The top number of a fraction is called the **numerator**, and it represents the number of parts under consideration. The 1 in $\frac{1}{4}$ means that 1 part out of the whole is being considered in the calculation.

The bottom number of a fraction is called the **denominator**, and it represents the total number of equal parts. The 4 in $\frac{1}{4}$ means that the whole consists of 4 equal parts.

It represents the **quotient** of the two numbers "x divided by y." It can also be thought of as x out of y equal parts.

What is an "undefined" fraction?

How can fractions be manipulated without changing the value of the fraction?

What are equivalent fractions?

Show how the following equivalent fractions can be reduced: $\frac{2}{10}, \frac{3}{15}, \frac{4}{20}$, and $\frac{5}{25}$.

What are proper fractions, improper fractions, and mixed numbers?

How can the improper fraction $\frac{8}{3}$ be rewritten as a mixed number?

Fractions can be manipulated, without changing the value of the fraction, by multiplying or dividing (but not adding or subtracting) both the numerator and denominator by the same number.

If you divide both numbers by a common factor, you are **reducing** or simplifying the fraction.

A fraction cannot have a denominator of zero; this is referred to as "*undefined*."

For example, $\frac{2}{10}, \frac{3}{15}, \frac{4}{20}$, and $\frac{5}{25}$ are all equivalent fractions. They can also all be reduced or simplified to $\frac{1}{5}$.

Two fractions that have the same value, but are expressed differently are known as **equivalent fractions**.

Any improper fraction can be rewritten as a mixed number. Example: $\frac{8}{3} = \frac{6}{3} + \frac{2}{3} = 2 + \frac{2}{3} = 2\frac{2}{3}$.

A fraction whose denominator is greater than its numerator is known as a **proper fraction**, while a fraction whose numerator is greater than its denominator is known as an **improper fraction**. Proper fractions have values *less than one* and improper fractions have values *greater than one*.

A **mixed number** is a number that contains both an integer and a fraction.

Numbers and Operations
ATI TEAS Mathematics

How can the mixed number $1\frac{3}{5}$ be rewritten as an improper fraction?

Numbers and Operations
ATI TEAS Mathematics

What is one way for a model to represent the decimal 0.24?

Numbers and Operations
ATI TEAS Mathematics

How can 0.24 be written as a fraction?

Numbers and Operations
ATI TEAS Mathematics

What are percentages?

Numbers and Operations
ATI TEAS Mathematics

How can fractions be expressed as percents?

Numbers and Operations
ATI TEAS Mathematics

What would $\frac{7}{10}$ and $\frac{1}{4}$ be as percentages?

The decimal 0.24 is twenty four hundredths. One possible model to represent this fraction is to draw 100 pennies, since each penny is worth 1 one hundredth of a dollar. Draw one hundred circles to represent one hundred pennies. Shade 24 of the pennies to represent the decimal twenty-four hundredths.

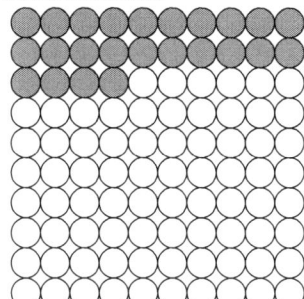

Percentages can be thought of as fractions that are based on a whole of 100; that is, one whole is equal to 100%. The word percent means "per hundred."

Example:

$$\frac{7}{10} = \frac{70}{100} = 70\%$$

$$\frac{1}{4} = \frac{25}{100} = 25\%$$

Any mixed number can be rewritten as an improper fraction. Example: $1\frac{3}{5} = 1 + \frac{3}{5} = \frac{5}{5} + \frac{3}{5} = \frac{8}{5}$.

To write the decimal as a fraction, write a fraction: $\frac{\# \ shaded \ spaces}{\# \ total \ spaces}$. The number of shaded spaces is 24, and the total number of spaces is 100, so as a fraction 0.24 equals $\frac{24}{100}$. This fraction can then be reduced to $\frac{6}{25}$.

Fractions can be expressed as percents by finding equivalent fractions with a denomination of 100.

How can you express a percentage as a fraction?

What would 60% and 96% be as fractions?

How do you convert from a decimal to a percent and a percent to decimal?

What are .23, 5.34, and .007 written as percentages?

What are 700%, 86%, and .15% written as decimals?

How can 15% be written as a fraction?

Example:

$$60\% = \frac{60}{100} = \frac{3}{5}$$

$$96\% = \frac{96}{100} = \frac{24}{25}$$

To express a percentage as a fraction, divide the percentage number by 100 and reduce the fraction to its simplest possible terms.

0.23 = 23%

5.34 = 534%

0.007 = 0.7%

Converting decimals to percentages and percentages to decimals is as simple as moving the decimal point.

To *convert from a decimal to a percent*, move the decimal point **two places to the right**.

To *convert from a percent to a decimal*, move it **two places to the left**.

15% written as a fraction is $\frac{15}{100}$ which equals $\frac{3}{20}$.

To convert a percent to a fraction, follow these steps:

1) Write the percent over 100 because percent means "per one hundred." So, 15% can be written as $\frac{15}{100}$.

2) Fractions should be written in simplest form, which means that the numbers in the numerator and denominator should be reduced if possible. Both 15 and 100 can be divided by 5.

3) Therefore, $\frac{15 \div 5}{100 \div 5} = \frac{3}{20}$.

700% = 7.00

86% = 0.86

0.15% = 0.0015

It may be helpful to remember that the percentage number will always be larger than the equivalent decimal number.

How can 15% be written as a decimal?

How can 24.36% be written as a fraction and as a decimal?

How can $\frac{4}{5}$ be converted to a decimal and to a percent?

How can $3\frac{2}{5}$ be converted to a decimal and to a percent?

What is addition?

What is subtraction?

24.36% written as a fraction is $\frac{24.36}{100}$, or $\frac{2436}{10,000}$, which reduces to $\frac{609}{2500}$.

24.36% written as a decimal is 0.2436.

Recall that dividing by 100 moves the decimal two places to the left.

15% written as a decimal is 0.15.

To convert a percent to a decimal, follow these steps:

1) Write the percent over 100 because percent means "per one hundred." So, 15% can be written as $\frac{15}{100}$.

2) 15 divided by 100 equals 0.15, so 15% = 0.15. In other words, when converting from a percent to a decimal, drop the percent sign and move the decimal two places to the left.

The mixed number $3\frac{2}{5}$ has a whole number and a fractional part. The fractional part $\frac{2}{5}$ can be written as a decimal by dividing 5 into 2, which gives 0.4. Adding the whole to the part gives 3.4. Alternatively, note that $3\frac{2}{5} = 3\frac{4}{10} = 3.4$

To change a decimal to a percent, multiply it by 100. 3.4(100) = 340%. Notice that this percentage is greater than 100%. This makes sense because the original mixed number $3\frac{2}{5}$ is greater than 1.

To convert a fraction to a decimal, simply divide the numerator by the denominator in the fraction. The numerator is the top number in the fraction and the denominator is the bottom number in a fraction. So $\frac{4}{5} = 4 \div 5 = 0.80 = 0.8$.

Percent means "per hundred." $\frac{4 \times 20}{5 \times 20} = \frac{80}{100} = 80\%$.

Subtraction is the opposite operation to addition; it decreases the value of one quantity by the value of another quantity.
Example: $6 - 4 = 2; 17 - 8 = 9$.

The result is called the **difference**. Note that with subtraction, the order does matter. $6 - 4 \neq 4 - 6$.

Addition increases the value of one quantity by the value of another quantity. Example: $2 + 4 = 6; 8 + 9 = 17$. The result is called the **sum**.

With addition, the order does not matter. $4 + 2 = 2 + 4$.

What is multiplication?

What is division?

What is Order of Operations?

What is a helpful way to remember the steps of Order of Operations?

How can $5 + 20 \div 4 \times (2 + 3) - 6$ be solved with the Order of Operations?

What are parentheses?

Division is the opposite operation to multiplication; one number tells us how many parts to divide the other number into. Example: $20 \div 4 = 5$; if 20 is split into 4 equal parts, each part is 5. With division, the order of the numbers does matter. $20 \div 4 \neq 4 \div 20$.

Multiplication can be thought of as repeated addition. One number tells how many times to add the other number to itself. Example: 3×2 (three times two) $= 2 + 2 + 2 = 6$. With multiplication, the order does not matter. $2 \times 3 = 3 \times 2$ or $3 + 3 = 2 + 2 + 2$.

The most common mnemonic for the order of operations is **PEMDAS**, or "Please Excuse My Dear Aunt Sally." PEMDAS stands for parentheses, exponents, multiplication, division, addition, and subtraction. It is important to understand that multiplication and division have equal precedence, as do addition and subtraction, so those pairs of operations are simply worked from left to right in order.
Example: Evaluate the expression $5 + 20 \div 4 \times (2 + 3)^2 - 6$ using the correct order of operations.

- **P:** Perform the operations inside the parentheses: $(2 + 3) = 5$
- **E:** Simplify the exponents: $(5)^2 = 5 \times 5 = 25$
    - The expression now looks like this: $5 + 20 \div 4 \times 25 - 6$
- **MD:** Perform multiplication and division from left to right: $20 \div 4 = 5$; then $5 \times 25 = 125$
    - The expression now looks like this: $5 + 125 - 6$
- **AS:** Perform addition and subtraction from left to right: $5 + 125 = 130$; then $130 - 6 = 124$

The **order of operations** is a set of rules that dictates the order in which we must perform each operation in an expression so that we will evaluate it accurately. If we have an expression that includes multiple different operations, the order of operations tells us which operations to do first.

Parentheses are used to designate which operations should be done first when there are multiple operations.

P: Perform the operations inside the parentheses: $(2 + 3) = 5$

E: Simplify the exponents. (Not required on the ATI TEAS).
The equation now looks like this: $5 + 20 \div 4 \times 5 - 6$

MD: Perform multiplication and division from left to right: $20 \div 4 = 5$; then $5 \times 5 = 25$
The equation now looks like this: $5 + 25 - 6$

AS: Perform addition and subtraction from left to right: $5 + 25 = 30$; then $30 - 6 = 24$

Numbers and Operations
© Mometrix Media – flashcardsecrets.com/teas
ATI TEAS Mathematics

How should the equation 4 − (2 + 1) = 1 be solved?

Numbers and Operations
© Mometrix Media – flashcardsecrets.com/teas
ATI TEAS Mathematics

What is an exponent?

Numbers and Operations
© Mometrix Media – flashcardsecrets.com/teas
ATI TEAS Mathematics

What are squared and cubed exponents and negative exponents?

Numbers and Operations
© Mometrix Media – flashcardsecrets.com/teas
ATI TEAS Mathematics

Define *absolute value*.

Numbers and Operations
© Mometrix Media – flashcardsecrets.com/teas
ATI TEAS Mathematics

What needs to be done to show that $|3| = |-3|$?

Numbers and Operations
© Mometrix Media – flashcardsecrets.com/teas
ATI TEAS Mathematics

What needs to be done to add positive and negative numbers?

An **exponent** is a superscript number placed next to another number at the top right. It indicates how many times the base number is to be multiplied by itself. Exponents provide a shorthand way to write what would be a longer mathematical expression.

Example: $a^2 = a \times a$;

$2^4 = 2 \times 2 \times 2 \times 2$.

The parentheses tell us that we must add 2 and 1, and then subtract the sum from 4, rather than subtracting 2 from 4 and then adding 1 (this would give us an answer of 3).

A precursor to working with negative numbers is understanding what **absolute values** are. A number's *Absolute Value* is simply the distance away from zero a number is on the number line. The absolute value of a number is always positive and is written $|x|$.

A number with an exponent of 2 is said to be "squared," while a number with an exponent of 3 is said to be "cubed." The value of a number raised to an exponent is called its power.

So, 8^4 is read as "8 to the 4th power," or "8 raised to the power of 4."

A negative exponent is the same as the reciprocal of a positive exponent. Example: $a^{-2} = \frac{1}{a^2}$.

When adding signed numbers, if the signs are the same simply add the absolute values of the addends and apply the original sign to the sum. For example, $(+4) + (+8) = +12$ and $(-4) + (-8) = -12$.

When the original signs are different, take the absolute values of the addends and subtract the smaller value from the larger value, then apply the original sign of the larger value to the difference. For instance, $(+4) + (-8) = -4$ and $(-4) + (+8) = +4$.

The absolute value of 3, written as $|3|$, is 3 because the distance between 0 and 3 on a number line is three units. Likewise, the absolute value of –3, written as $|-3|$, is 3 because the distance between 0 and –3 on a number line is three units. So, $|3| = |-3|$.

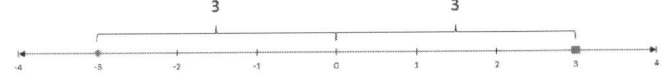

Numbers and Operations

What needs to be done to subtract positive and negative numbers?

Numbers and Operations

What needs to be done to multiply positive and negative numbers?

Numbers and Operations

What needs to be done to divide positive and negative numbers?

Numbers and Operations

What needs to be done to add and subtract decimals?

Numbers and Operations

What needs to be done to multiply decimals?

Numbers and Operations

How can you multiply 12.3 and 2.56?

If the signs are the same the product is positive when multiplying signed numbers. For example, $(+4) \times (+8) = +32$ and $(-4) \times (-8) = +32$.

If the signs are opposite, the product is negative. For example, $(+4) \times (-8) = -32$ and $(-4) \times (+8) = -32$.

When more than two factors are multiplied together, the sign of the product is determined by how many negative factors are present.

If there are an odd number of negative factors then the product is negative, whereas an even number of negative factors indicates a positive product. For instance, $(+4) \times (-8) \times (-2) = +64$ and $(-4) \times (-8) \times (-2) = -64$.

For subtracting signed numbers, change the sign of the number after the minus symbol and then follow the same rules used for addition. For example, $(+4) - (+8) = (+4) + (-8) = -4$.

When adding and subtracting decimals, the decimal points must always be aligned. Adding decimals is just like adding regular whole numbers. Example: $4.5 + 2 = 6.5$.

An easy way to add decimals is to align all of the decimal points in a vertical column visually. This will allow you to see exactly where the decimal should be placed in the final answer. Begin adding from right to left. Add each column in turn, making sure to carry the number to the left if a column adds up to more than 9.

The same rules apply to the subtraction of decimals.

The rules for dividing signed numbers are similar to multiplying signed numbers. If the dividend and divisor have the same sign, the quotient is positive. If the dividend and divisor have opposite signs, the quotient is negative. For example, $(-4) \div (+8) = -0.5$.

For example, 12.3×2.56 has three places to the right of the respective decimals. Multiply 123×256 to get 31488. Now, beginning on the right, count three places to the left and insert the decimal. The final product will be 31.488.

A simple multiplication problem has two components: a **multiplicand** and a **multiplier**. When multiplying decimals, work as though the numbers were whole rather than decimals.

Once the final product is calculated, count the number of places to the right of the decimal in both the multiplicand and the multiplier. Then, count that number of places from the right of the product and place the decimal in that position.

Numbers and Operations

What needs to be done to divide decimals?

Numbers and Operations

How can you divide 4.9 and 24.5?

Numbers and Operations

What needs to be done to add and subtract fractions?

Numbers and Operations

What needs to be done to multiply fractions?

Numbers and Operations

What needs to be done to divide fractions?

Numbers and Operations

What is a number line?

For example, 4.9 into 24.5 would become 49 into 245. The decimal was moved one space to the right to create a whole number in the divisor, and then the same was done for the dividend. Once the whole numbers are created, the problem is carried out normally: 245 ÷ 49 = 5.

Every division problem has a **divisor** and a **dividend**. The dividend is the number that is being divided. In the problem 14 ÷ 7, 14 is the dividend and 7 is the divisor. In a division problem with decimals, the divisor must be converted into a whole number.

Begin by moving the decimal in the divisor to the right until a whole number is created. Next, move the decimal in the dividend the same number of spaces to the right.

Two fractions can be multiplied by multiplying the two numerators to find the new numerator and the two denominators to find the new denominator.

Example: $\frac{1}{3} \times \frac{2}{3} = \frac{1 \times 2}{3 \times 3} = \frac{2}{9}$.

If two fractions have a common denominator, they can be added or subtracted simply by adding or subtracting the two numerators and retaining the same denominator.

Example: $\frac{1}{2} + \frac{1}{4} = \frac{2}{4} + \frac{1}{4} = \frac{3}{4}$.

If the two fractions do not already have the same denominator, one or both of them must be manipulated to achieve a common denominator before they can be added or subtracted.

A **number line** is a graph to see the distance between numbers. Basically, this graph shows the relationship between numbers.

So, a number line may have a point for zero and may show negative numbers on the left side of the line. Also, any positive numbers are placed on the right side of the line.

Two fractions can be divided by flipping the numerator and denominator of the second fraction and then proceeding as though it were a multiplication.

Example: $\frac{2}{3} \div \frac{3}{4} = \frac{2}{3} \times \frac{4}{3} = \frac{8}{9}$.

Numbers and Operations
© Mometrix Media – flashcardsecrets.com/teas
ATI TEAS Mathematics

What is the value of each point on the number line below?

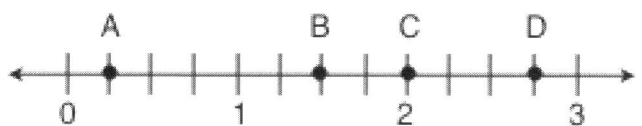

Numbers and Operations
© Mometrix Media – flashcardsecrets.com/teas
ATI TEAS Mathematics

What is the order the following rational numbers from least to greatest: $0.55, 17\%, \sqrt{25}, \frac{64}{4}, \frac{25}{50}, 3$?

Numbers and Operations
© Mometrix Media – flashcardsecrets.com/teas
ATI TEAS Mathematics

What is the order the following rational numbers from greatest to least:
$0.3, 27\%, \sqrt{100}, \frac{72}{9}, \frac{1}{9}, 4.5$

Numbers and Operations
© Mometrix Media – flashcardsecrets.com/teas
ATI TEAS Mathematics

How can you find the common denominator of two fractions?

Numbers and Operations
© Mometrix Media – flashcardsecrets.com/teas
ATI TEAS Mathematics

What are factors and common factors?

Numbers and Operations
© Mometrix Media – flashcardsecrets.com/teas
ATI TEAS Mathematics

What are prime factors and greatest common factors?

Recall that the term **rational** simply means that the number can be expressed as a ratio or fraction. The set of rational numbers includes integers and decimals. Notice that each of the numbers in the problem can be written as a decimal or integer:

17% = 0.17

$\sqrt{25} = 5$

$\frac{64}{4} = 16$

$\frac{25}{50} = \frac{1}{2} = 0.5$

So, the answer is 17%, $\frac{25}{50}$, 0.55, 3, $\sqrt{25}$, $\frac{64}{4}$.

Use the dashed lines on the number line to identify each point. Each dashed line between two whole numbers is $\frac{1}{4}$. The line halfway between two numbers is $\frac{1}{2}$.

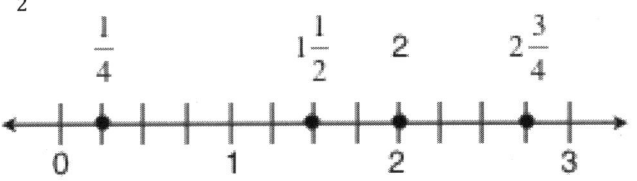

When two fractions are manipulated so that they have the same denominator, this is known as finding a **common denominator**. The number chosen to be that common denominator should be the **least common multiple** of the two original denominators.

Example: $\frac{3}{4}$ and $\frac{5}{6}$; the least common multiple of 4 and 6 is 12. Manipulating to achieve the common denominator: $\frac{3}{4} = \frac{9}{12}$; $\frac{5}{6} = \frac{10}{12}$.

Recall that the term **rational** simply means that the number can be expressed as a ratio or fraction. The set of rational numbers includes integers and decimals. Notice that each of the numbers in the problem can be written as a decimal or integer:

27% = 0.27

$\sqrt{100} = 10$

$\frac{72}{9} = 8$

$\frac{1}{9} \approx 0.11$

So, the answer is $\sqrt{100}$, $\frac{72}{9}$, 4.5, 0.3, 27%, $\frac{1}{9}$.

A **prime factor** is also a prime number. Therefore, the prime factors of 12 are 2 and 3. For 15, the prime factors are 3 and 5.

The **greatest common factor (GCF)** is the largest number that is a factor of two or more numbers. For example, the factors of 15 are 1, 3, 5, and 15; the factors of 35 are 1, 5, 7, and 35. Therefore, the greatest common factor of 15 and 35 is 5.

Factors are numbers that are multiplied together to obtain a **product**. For example, in the equation $2 \times 3 = 6$, the numbers 2 and 3 are factors. A **prime number** has only two factors (1 and itself), but other numbers can have many factors.

A **common factor** is a number that divides exactly into two or more other numbers. For example, the factors of 12 are 1, 2, 3, 4, 6, and 12, while the factors of 15 are 1, 3, 5, and 15. The common factors of 12 and 15 are 1 and 3.

What are multiples and least common multiples?

How can manipulate equations in order to find the missing variable?

Ray earns $10 an hour. Now, let's say that Ray makes $360. How many hours did he work to make $360?

Describe *one variable linear equations*, and give the name of the solutions to those equations.

What needs to be done to find the solution to $5x + 10 = 0$?

$\frac{45\%}{12\%} = \frac{15\%}{x}$. Solve for x.

Sometimes you will have variables missing in equations. So, you need to find the missing variable. To do this, you need to remember one important thing: *whatever you do to one side of an equation, you need to do to the other side.*

If you subtract 100 from one side of an equation, you need to subtract 100 from the other side of the equation. This will allow you to change the form of the equation to find missing values.

The **least common multiple** (**LCM**) is the smallest number that is a multiple of two or more numbers.

For example, the multiples of 3 include 3, 6, 9, 12, 15, etc.; the multiples of 5 include 5, 10, 15, 20, etc.

Therefore, the least common multiple of 3 and 5 is 15.

Another way to write an equation is $ax + b = 0$ where $a \neq 0$. This is known as a **one-variable linear equation**.

A solution to an equation is called a **root**.

Ray's wages can be calculated with the equation $y = 10x$, where y is his wages and x is the number of hours that he works. The independent variable is x; this is the variable that drives the other variable. The dependent variable is y; this is the variable that changes based on the other variable.

Now, you want to know how many hours Ray worked to earn \$360. To do this, set up the equation with \$360 substituted for y: $\$360 = 10x$. You want to find the value for x, so divide both sides of the equation by 10:

$$\frac{360}{10} = \frac{10x}{10}$$

So you have $x = 36$. Ray worked 36 hours to make \$360.

First, cross multiply; then, solve for x: $\frac{45\%}{12\%} = \frac{15\%}{x}$

$\frac{0.45}{0.12} = \frac{0.15}{x}$

$0.45(x) = 0.12(0.15)$
$0.45x = 0.0180$
$0.45x \div 0.45 = 0.0180 \div 0.45$
$x = 0.04 = 4\%$

Alternatively, notice that $\frac{45\% \div 3}{12\% \div 3} = \frac{15\%}{4\%}$. So, $x = 4\%$.

If we solve for x, the solution is $x = -2$. In other words, the root of the equation is –2.
The first step is to subtract 10 from both sides. This gives $5x = -10$.

Next, divide both sides by the **coefficient** of the variable. For this example, that is 5. So, you should have $x = -2$.

You can make sure that you have the correct answer by placing –2 back into the original equation. So, the equation now looks like this: $(5)(-2) + 10 = -10 + 10 = 0$.

Numbers and Operations
ATI TEAS Mathematics

How do you solve for x in the proportion $\frac{0.50}{2} = \frac{1.50}{x}$?

Numbers and Operations
ATI TEAS Mathematics

$\frac{40}{8} = \frac{x}{24}$. Find x.

Numbers and Operations
ATI TEAS Mathematics

Demonstrate how to subtract 189 from 525 using regrouping. You can start by setting up the subtraction problem as:

$$\begin{array}{r} 525 \\ -\ 189 \\ \hline \end{array}$$

Numbers and Operations
ATI TEAS Mathematics

Demonstrate how to subtract 477 from 620 using regrouping. You can start by setting up the subtraction problem as:

$$\begin{array}{r} 620 \\ -\ 477 \\ \hline \end{array}$$

Numbers and Operations
ATI TEAS Mathematics

A patient's age is thirteen more than half of 60. How old is the patient?

Numbers and Operations
ATI TEAS Mathematics

A patient was given pain medicine at a dosage of 0.22 grams. The patient's dosage was then increased to 0.80 grams. By how much was the patient's dosage increased?

One way to solve for x is to first cross multiply.
$\frac{40}{8} = \frac{x}{24}$.

$40(24) = 8(x)$
$960 = 8x$
$960 \div 8 = 8x \div 8$
$x = 120$

Or, notice that:
$\frac{40 \times 3}{8 \times 3} = \frac{120}{24}$, so $x = 120$

First, cross multiply; then, solve for x.
$\frac{0.50}{2} = \frac{1.50}{x}$.

$0.50(x) = 2(1.50)$
$0.50x = 3$
$0.50x \div 0.50 = 3 \div 0.50$
$x = 6$

Or, notice that $\frac{0.50 \times 3}{2 \times 3} = \frac{1.50}{6}$, so $x = 6$.

Notice that the numbers in the ones and tens columns of 620 are smaller than the numbers in the ones and tens columns of 477. This means you will need to use regrouping to perform subtraction.

```
   6  2  0
-  4  7  7
```

To subtract 7 from 0 in the ones column you will need to borrow from the 2 in the tens column.

```
   6  1  10
-  4  7   7
           3
```

Next, to subtract 7 from the 1 that's still in the tens column you will need to borrow from the 6 in the hundreds column.

```
   5  11  10
-  4   7   7
       4   3
```

Lastly, subtract 4 from the 5 remaining in the hundreds column to get:

```
   5  11  10
-  4   7   7
   1   4   3
```

Notice that the numbers in the ones and tens columns of 525 are smaller than the numbers in the ones and tens columns of 189. This means you will need to use regrouping to perform subtraction.

```
   5  2  5
-  1  8  9
```

To subtract 9 from 5 in the ones column you will need to borrow from the 2 in the tens columns:

```
   5  1  15
-  1  8   9
          6
```

Next, to subtract 8 from 1 in the tens column you will need to borrow from the 5 in the hundreds column:

```
   4  11  15
-  1   8   9
       3   6
```

Last, subtract the 1 from the 4 in the hundreds column:

```
   4  11  15
-  1   8   9
   3   3   6
```

The first step is to determine what operation (addition, subtraction, multiplication, or division) the problem requires. Notice the key words and phrases "by how much" and "increased." "Increased" means that you go from a smaller amount to a larger amount. This change can be found by subtracting the smaller amount from the larger amount: 0.80 grams – 0.22 grams = 0.58 grams.

Remember to line up the decimal when subtracting.
```
   0.80
-  0.22
   0.58
```

"More than" indicates addition, and "of" indicates multiplication. The expression can be written as $\frac{1}{2}(60) + 13$.

So, the patient's age is equal to $\frac{1}{2}(60) + 13 = 30 + 13 = 43$. The patient is 43 years old.

Numbers and Operations
© Mometrix Media – flashcardsecrets.com/teas
ATI TEAS Mathematics

At a hospital, $\frac{3}{4}$ of the 100 beds are occupied today. Yesterday, $\frac{4}{5}$ of the 100 beds were occupied. On which day were more of the hospital beds occupied and by how much more?

Numbers and Operations
© Mometrix Media – flashcardsecrets.com/teas
ATI TEAS Mathematics

At a hospital, 40% of the nurses work in labor and delivery. If 20 nurses work in labor and delivery, how many nurses work at the hospital?

Numbers and Operations
© Mometrix Media – flashcardsecrets.com/teas
ATI TEAS Mathematics

A patient was given blood pressure medicine at a dosage of 2 grams. The patient's dosage was then decreased to 0.45 grams. By how much was the patient's dosage decreased?

Numbers and Operations
© Mometrix Media – flashcardsecrets.com/teas
ATI TEAS Mathematics

Two weeks ago, $\frac{2}{3}$ of the 60 patients at a hospital were male. Last week, $\frac{3}{6}$ of the 80 patients were male. During which week were there more male patients?

Numbers and Operations
© Mometrix Media – flashcardsecrets.com/teas
ATI TEAS Mathematics

Jane ate lunch at a local restaurant. She ordered a $4.99 appetizer, a $12.50 entrée, and a $1.25 soda. If she wants to tip her server 20%, how much money will she spend in all?

Numbers and Operations
© Mometrix Media – flashcardsecrets.com/teas
ATI TEAS Mathematics

What are the three main ways that a percentage problem can be presented?

To answer this problem, first think about the number of nurses that work at the hospital. Will it be more or less than the number of nurses who work in a specific department such as labor and delivery? More nurses work at the hospital, so the number you find to answer this question will be greater than 20.

40% of the nurses are labor and delivery nurses. "Of" indicates multiplication, and words like "is" and "are" indicate equivalence. Translating the problem into a mathematical sentence gives $40\% \times n = 20$, where n represents the total number of nurses. Solving for n gives $n = \frac{20}{40\%} = \frac{20}{0.40} = 50$.

Fifty nurses work at the hospital.

First, find the actual number of beds that were occupied each day. To do so, multiply the fraction of beds occupied by the number of beds available:
Actual number of beds occupied = fraction of beds occupied × number of beds available
Today: Actual number of beds occupied = $\frac{3}{4} \times 100$.
$\frac{3}{4} \times \frac{100}{1} = \frac{3 \times 100}{4 \times 1} = \frac{300}{4}$
Then, write the fraction in lowest terms. $\frac{300}{4} \div \frac{4}{4} = \frac{75}{1} = 75$.
Today, 75 beds are occupied.
Yesterday: Actual number of beds occupied = $\frac{4}{5} \times 100$.
$\frac{4}{5} \times \frac{100}{1} = \frac{4 \times 100}{5 \times 1} = \frac{400}{5}$
Then, write the fraction in lowest terms. $\frac{400}{5} \div \frac{5}{5} = \frac{80}{1} = 80$.
Yesterday, 80 beds were occupied.
The difference in the number of beds occupied is 80 − 75 = 5 beds.
Therefore, five more beds were occupied yesterday than today.

First, you need to find the number of male patients that were in the hospital each week. You are given this amount in terms of fractions. To find the actual number of male patients, multiply the fraction of male patients by the number of patients in the hospital.
Actual number of male patients = fraction of male patients × total number of patients.

Two weeks ago: Actual number of male patients = $\frac{2}{3} \times 60$.
$\frac{2}{3} \times \frac{60}{1} = \frac{2 \times 60}{3 \times 1} = \frac{120}{3} = 40$.
Two weeks ago, 40 of the patients were male.
Last week: Actual number of male patients = $\frac{3}{6} \times 80$.
$\frac{3}{6} \times \frac{80}{1} = \frac{3 \times 80}{6 \times 1} = \frac{240}{6} = 40$.

Last week, 40 of the patients were male.
The number of male patients was the same both weeks.

The decrease is represented by the difference between the two amounts:
2 grams − 0.45 grams = 1.55 grams.
Remember to line up the decimal point before subtracting.
```
   2.00
-  0.45
   1.55
```

A percentage problem can be presented three main ways:
Type (1) Find what percentage of some number another number is. Example: What percentage of 40 is 8?

Type (2) Find what number is some percentage of a given number. Example: What number is 20% of 40?

Type (3) Find what number another number is a given percentage of. Example: What number is 8 20% of?

To find total amount, first find the sum of the items she ordered from the menu and then add 20% of this sum to the total.

In other words:
$4.99 + $12.50 + $1.25 = $18.74.
Then 20% of $18.74 is (20%)($18.74) = (0.20)($18.74) = $3.75.

So, the total she spends is cost of the meal plus the tip or $18.74 + $3.75 = $22.49.

Another way to find this sum is to multiply 120% by the cost of the meal.
$18.74(120%) = $18.74(1.20) = $22.49.

Numbers and Operations
ATI TEAS Mathematics

What are the forms used to solve each type of percentage problem?

Numbers and Operations
ATI TEAS Mathematics

In a school cafeteria, 7 students choose pizza, 9 choose hamburgers, and 4 choose tacos. Find the percentage that chooses tacos.

Numbers and Operations
ATI TEAS Mathematics

What is 30% of 120?

Numbers and Operations
ATI TEAS Mathematics

What is 150% of 20?

Numbers and Operations
ATI TEAS Mathematics

What is 14.5% of 96?

Numbers and Operations
ATI TEAS Mathematics

According to a hospital survey, 82% of nurses were highly satisfied at their job. Of 145 nurses, how many were highly satisfied?

The thing that frequently makes percentage problems difficult is that they are most often also word problems, so a large part of solving them is figuring out which quantities are what.

To find the whole, you must first add all of the parts: $7 + 9 + 4 = 20$. The percentage can then be found by dividing the part by the whole $\left(\% = \frac{P}{W}\right)$: $\frac{4}{20} = \frac{20}{100} = 20\%$.

The three components in all of these cases are the same: a **whole** (W), a **part** (P), and a **percentage** (%).

These are related by the equation: $\boldsymbol{P = W \times \%}$. This is the form of the equation you would use to solve problems of type (2).

To solve types (1) and (3), you would use these two forms: $\% = \frac{P}{W}$ and $W = \frac{P}{\%}$

150% of 20 is found by multiplying 150% by 20. First, change 150% to a fraction or decimal. Recall that "percent" means per hundred, so $150\% = \frac{150}{100} = 1.50$.

So, $(1.50)(20) = 30$. Notice that 30 is greater than the original number of 20. This makes sense because you are finding a number that is more than 100% of the original number.

The word "of" indicates multiplication, so 30% of 120 is found by multiplying 30% by 120. First, change 30% to a fraction or decimal.

Recall that "percent" means per hundred, so $30\% = \frac{30}{100} = 0.30$. 120 times 0.3 is 36.

82% of 145 = 0.82 × 145 = 118.9.

Because you can't have 0.9 of a person, the answer is "about 119 nurses are highly satisfied with their jobs."

Change 14.5% to a decimal before multiplying. 0.145 × 96 = 13.92.

Notice that 13.92 is much smaller than the original number of 96. This makes sense because you are finding a small percentage of the original number.

A patient was given 40 mg of a certain medicine. Later, the patient's dosage was increased to 45 mg. What was the percent increase in his medication?

A patient was given 100 mg of a certain medicine. The patient's dosage was later decreased to 88 mg. What was the percent decrease?

What is rounding?

Round each number to the nearest ten: 11, 47, 118.

Round each number to the nearest hundred: 78, 980, 248.

Round each number to the nearest thousand: 302, 1274, 3756.

The medication was decreased by 12 mg (100 mg – 88 mg = 12 mg). To find by what percent the medication was decreased, this change must be written as a percentage when compared to the original amount. In other words, $\frac{\text{original amount} - \text{new amount}}{\text{original amount}} \times 100\% =$ percent decrease

So $\frac{12 \text{ mg}}{100 \text{ mg}} \times 100\% = 0.12 \times 100\% = 12\%$.
The percent decrease is 12%.

To find the percent increase, first compare the original and increased amounts. The original amount was 40 mg, and the increased amount is 45 mg, so the dosage of medication was increased by 5 mg (45 – 40 = 5). Note, however, that the question asks not by how much the dosage increased but by what percentage it increased.

Percent increase = $\frac{\text{new amount} - \text{original amount}}{\text{original amount}} \times 100\%$.

So, $\frac{45 \text{ mg} - 40 \text{ mg}}{40 \text{ mg}} \times 100\% = \frac{5}{40} \times 100\% = 0.125 \times 100\% = 12.5\%$
The percent increase is 12.5%.

Remember, when rounding to the nearest ten, anything ending in 5 or greater rounds up. So, 11 rounds to 10, 47 rounds to 50, and 118 rounds to 120

Rounding is reducing the digits in a number while still trying to keep the value similar. The result will be less accurate but in a simpler form and easier to use. Whole numbers can be rounded to the nearest ten, hundred, or thousand.

Remember, when rounding to the nearest thousand, anything ending in 500 or greater rounds up. So, 302 rounds to 0, 1274 rounds to 1000, and 3756 rounds to 4000.

Remember, when rounding to the nearest hundred, anything ending in 50 or greater rounds up. So, 78 rounds to 100, 980 rounds to 1000, and 248 rounds to 200.

What is estimation?

Estimate the solution to: 345,932 + 96,369.

A patient's heart beat 422 times over the course of six minutes. About how many times did the patient's heart beat during each minute?

Define *proportion* and *direct proportion*, and give an example of a directly proportional relationship.

Define *inverse proportion*, and give an example of an inversely proportional relationship.

What is a ratio?

Start by rounding each number to have only one digit as a non-zero number: 345,932 becomes 300,000 and 96,369 becomes 100,000.

Then, add the rounded numbers: 300,000 + 100,000 = 400,000. So, the answer is approximately 400,000.

The exact answer would be 345,932 + 96,369 = 442,301. So, the estimate of 400,000 is a similar value to the exact answer.

When you are asked for the solution a problem, you may need to provide only an approximate figure or **estimation** for your answer.

In this situation, you can round the numbers that will be calculated to a non-zero number. This means that the first digit in the number is not zero, and the following numbers are zeros.

A proportion is a relationship between two quantities that dictates how one changes when the other changes.

A **direct proportion** describes a relationship in which a quantity increases by a set amount for every increase in the other quantity, or decreases by that same amount for every decrease in the other quantity.

Example: Assuming a constant driving speed, the time required for a car trip increases as the distance of the trip increases. The distance to be traveled and the time required to travel are directly proportional.

"About how many" indicates that you need to estimate the solution. In this case, look at the numbers you are given. 422 can be rounded down to 420, which is easily divisible by 6.

A good estimate is 420 ÷ 6 = 70 beats per minute. More accurately, the patient's heart rate was just over 70 beats per minute since his heart actually beat a little more than 420 times in six minutes.

A **ratio** is a comparison of two quantities in a particular order.

An **inverse proportion** is a relationship in which an increase in one quantity is accompanied by a decrease in the other, or vice versa.

Example: The time required for a car trip decreases as the speed increases, and increases as the speed decreases, so the time required is inversely proportional to the speed of the car.

There are 14 computers in a lab, and the class has 20 students. What is the student to computer ratio?

A patient was given 100 mg of a medicine every two hours. How much medication will the patient receive in four hours?

At a hospital, for every 20 female patients there are 15 male patients. This same patient ratio happens to exist at another hospital. If there are 100 female patients at the second hospital, how many male patients are there?

In a hospital emergency room, there are 4 nurses for every 12 patients. What is the ratio of nurses to patients? If the nurse-to-patient ratio remains constant, how many nurses must be present to care for 24 patients?

In an intensive care unit, the nurse-to-patient ratio is 1:2. If seven nurses are on duty, how many patients are currently in the ICU?

What is a constant of proportionality?

Using proportional reasoning, since four hours is twice as long as two hours, the patient will receive twice as much medication, 2 × 100 mg = 200 mg, within that time period. To write an equation, first, write the amount of medicine per 2 hours as a ratio.

$$\frac{100 \text{ mg}}{2 \text{ hours}}$$

Next create a proportion to relate the different time increments of 2 hours and 4 hours.

$\frac{100 \text{ mg}}{2 \text{ hours}} = \frac{x \text{ mg}}{4 \text{ hours}}$, where x is the amount of medicine the patient receives in four hours. Make sure to keep the same units in either the numerator or denominator. In this case the numerator units must be mg for both ratios and the denominator units must be hours for both ratios.

Use cross multiplication and division to solve for x.

$$\frac{100 \text{ mg}}{2 \text{ hours}} = \frac{x \text{ mg}}{4 \text{ hours}}$$

100(4) = 2(x) | 400 = 2x | 400 ÷ 2 = 2x ÷ 2 | 200 = x

Therefore, the patient receives 200 mg every four hours.

If there are 14 computers in a lab, and the class has 20 students, there is a student to computer ratio of 20 to 14, commonly written as 20:14.

Ratios are normally reduced to their smallest whole number representation, so 20:14 would be reduced to 10:7 by dividing both sides by 2.

The ratio of nurses to patients can be written as 4 to 12, 4:12, or $\frac{4}{12}$. Because four and twelve have a common factor of four, the ratio should be reduced to 1:3, which means that there is one nurse present for every three patients.

If this ratio remains constant, there must be eight nurses present to care for 24 patients.

One way to find the number of male patients is to set up and solve a proportion.

$$\frac{\text{number of female patients}}{\text{number of male patients}} = \frac{20}{15} = \frac{100}{\text{number of male patients}}.$$

Represent the unknown number of male patients as the variable x.

$$\frac{20}{15} = \frac{100}{x}.$$

Follow these steps to solve for x:
1. Cross multiply. $20 \times x = 15 \times 100$.
$20x = 1500$
2. Divide each side of the equation by 20.
$x = 75$

Or, notice that
$\frac{20 \times 5}{15 \times 5} = \frac{100}{75}$, so $x = 75$.

When two quantities have a proportional relationship, there exists a **constant of proportionality** between the quantities. The product of this constant and one of the quantities is equal to the other quantity.

Use proportional reasoning or set up a proportion to solve. Because there are twice as many patients as nurses, there must be fourteen patients when seven nurses are on duty. Setting up and solving a proportion gives the same result:

$$\frac{\text{number of nurses}}{\text{number of patients}} = \frac{1}{2} = \frac{7}{\text{number of patients}}$$

Represent the unknown number of customers as the variable x.

$$\frac{1}{2} = \frac{7}{x}$$

To solve for x, cross multiply:
$1 \times x = 7 \times 2$, so $x = 14$.

Numbers and Operations
© Mometrix Media – flashcardsecrets.com/teas
ATI TEAS Mathematics

If one lemon costs $0.25, two lemons cost $0.50, and three lemons cost $0.75, what is the constant of proportionality?

Numbers and Operations
© Mometrix Media – flashcardsecrets.com/teas
ATI TEAS Mathematics

How is slope found on a graph?

Numbers and Operations
© Mometrix Media – flashcardsecrets.com/teas
ATI TEAS Mathematics

What is the slope of the following chart?

# of Months on Sale	1	2	3	4	5
# of Copies Sold (In Thousands)	5	10	15	20	25

Numbers and Operations
© Mometrix Media – flashcardsecrets.com/teas
ATI TEAS Mathematics

What is unit rate?

Numbers and Operations
© Mometrix Media – flashcardsecrets.com/teas
ATI TEAS Mathematics

If you travel 30 miles every two hours, what is your unit rate?

Numbers and Operations
© Mometrix Media – flashcardsecrets.com/teas
ATI TEAS Mathematics

What are some common examples of unit rate?

On a graph with two points, (x_1, y_1) and (x_2, y_2), the **slope** is found with the formula $m = \frac{y_2 - y_1}{x_2 - x_1}$; where $x_1 \neq x_2$ and m stands for slope. If the value of the slope is **positive**, the line has an *upward direction* from left to right. If the value of the slope is **negative**, the line has a *downward direction* from left to right.

Unit rate expresses a quantity of one thing in terms of one unit of another.

Other examples are how much one ounce of food costs (price per ounce), or figuring out how much one egg costs out of the dozen (price per 1 egg, instead of price per 12 eggs). The denominator of a unit rate is always 1.

For example, if one lemon costs $0.25, two lemons cost $0.50, and three lemons cost $0.75, there is a proportional relationship between the total cost of lemons and the number of lemons purchased.

The constant of proportionality is the **unit price**, namely $0.25/lemon.

Notice that the total price of lemons, t, can be found by multiplying the unit price of lemons, p, and the number of lemons, n: $t = pn$.

So, the number of copies that are sold and the time that the book is on sale is a proportional relationship. In this example, an equation can be used to show the data: $y = 5x$, where x is the number of months that the book is on sale, and y is the number of copies sold. So, the slope is $\frac{rse}{run} = \frac{5}{1}$. This can be reduced to 5.

If you travel 30 miles every two hours, a unit rate expresses this comparison in terms of one hour: in one hour you travel 15 miles, so your unit rate is 15 miles per hour.

Soda #1 costs $1.50 for a 1-liter bottle, and soda #2 costs $2.75 for a 2-liter bottle. Which is the better deal?

If you can paint 2 rooms in 4.5 hours, how long it will take you to paint 5 rooms?

Janice made $40 during the first 5 hours she spent babysitting. She will continue to earn money at this rate until she finishes babysitting in 3 more hours. Find how much money Janice earned babysitting and how much she earns per hour.

The McDonalds are taking a family road trip, driving 300 miles to their cabin. It took them 2 hours to drive the first 120 miles. They will drive at the same speed all the way to their cabin. Find the speed at which the McDonalds are driving and how much longer it will take them to get to their cabin.

It takes Andy 10 minutes to read 6 pages of his book. He has already read 150 pages in his book that is 210 pages long. Find how long it takes Andy to read 1 page and also find how long it will take him to finish his book if he continues to read at the same speed.

What are the meanings of the following symbols that are used for inequalities (= | > | ≥ | < | ≤)?

Unit rates can also help determine the length of time a given event will take.

For example, if you can paint 2 rooms in 4.5 hours, you can determine how long it will take you to paint 5 rooms by solving for the unit rate per room and then multiplying that by 5.

Unit rates are used to compare different situations to solve problems. For example, to make sure you get the best deal when deciding which kind of soda to buy, you can find the unit rate of each.

If Soda #1 costs $1.50 for a 1-liter bottle, and soda #2 costs $2.75 for a 2-liter bottle, it would be a better deal to buy Soda #2, because its unit rate is only $1.375 per 1-liter, which is cheaper than Soda #1.

The McDonalds are driving 60 miles per hour. This can be found by setting up a proportion to find the unit rate, the number of miles they drive per one hour: $\frac{120}{2} = \frac{x}{1}$. Cross-multiplying yields $2x = 120$ and division by 2 shows that $x = 60$.

Since the McDonalds will drive this same speed for the remaining miles, it will take them another 3 hours to get to their cabin. This can be found by first finding how many miles the McDonalds have left to drive, which is 300 − 120 = 180. The McDonalds are driving at 60 miles per hour, so a proportion can be set up to determine how many hours it will take them to drive 180 miles: $\frac{180}{x} = \frac{60}{1}$. Cross-multiplying yields $60x = 180$, and division by 60 shows that $x = 3$. This can also be found by using the formula $D = r \times t$ (or $Distance = rate \times time$), where $180 = 60 \times t$, and division by 60 shows that $t = 3$.

Janice will earn $64 babysitting in her 8 total hours (adding the first 5 hours to the remaining 3 gives the 8 hour total). This can be found by setting up a proportion comparing money earned to babysitting hours. Since she earns $40 for 5 hours and since the rate is constant, she will earn a proportional amount in 8 hours: $\frac{40}{5} = \frac{x}{8}$. Cross-multiplying will yield $5x = 320$, and division by 5 shows that $x = 64$.

Janice earns $8 per hour. This can be found by taking her total amount earned, $64, and dividing it by the total number of hours worked, 8. Since $\frac{64}{8} = 8$, Janice makes $8 in one hour. This can also be found by finding the unit rate, money earned per hour: $\frac{64}{8} = \frac{x}{1}$. Since cross-multiplying yields $8x = 64$, and division by 8 shows that $x = 8$, Janice earns $8 per hour.

= equals, is equal to, is, was, were, will be, yields, is the same as, amounts to, becomes

> **is** greater than, **is** more than

≥ **is** greater than or equal to, is at least, is no less than

< **is** less than, **is** fewer than

≤ **is** less than or equal to, is at most, is no more than

It takes Andy 1 minute and 40 seconds to read one page in his book. This can be found by finding the unit rate per one page, by dividing the total time it takes him to read 6 pages by 6. Since it takes him 10 minutes to read 6 pages, $\frac{10}{6} = 1\frac{2}{3}$ minutes, which is 1 minute and 40 seconds.

It will take Andy another 100 minutes, or 1 hour and 40 minutes to finish his book. This can be found by first figuring out how many pages Andy has left to read, which is 210 − 150 = 60. Since it is now known that it takes him $1\frac{2}{3}$ minutes to read each page, then that rate must be multiplied by however many pages he has left to read (60) to find the time he'll need: $60 \times 1\frac{2}{3} = 100$, so it will take him 100 minutes, or 1 hour and 40 minutes, to read the rest of his book.

Numbers and Operations
© Mometrix Media – flashcardsecrets.com/teas
ATI TEAS Mathematics

How can you translate a sentence into an inequality?

Numbers and Operations
© Mometrix Media – flashcardsecrets.com/teas
ATI TEAS Mathematics

Translate the following paragraph to an inequality:
A farm sells vegetables and dairy products. One third of the sales from dairy products plus half of the sales from vegetables should be greater than the monthly payment (P) for the farm.

Numbers and Operations
© Mometrix Media – flashcardsecrets.com/teas
ATI TEAS Mathematics

Translate the following paragraph to a rational expression:
John and Luke play basketball every week. John can make 5 more shots per minute than Luke. On one day, John made 30 shots in the same time that it took Luke to make 20 shots. How fast are Luke and John making shots?

Numbers and Operations
© Mometrix Media – flashcardsecrets.com/teas
ATI TEAS Mathematics

Translate the following paragraph to a polynomial expression:
Fred buys some CDs for $12 each. He also buys two DVDs. The total that Fred spent is $60. So, write an equation that shows the connection between the number of CDs and the average cost of a DVD.

Numbers and Operations
© Mometrix Media – flashcardsecrets.com/teas
ATI TEAS Mathematics

What needs to be done to solve inequalities?

Numbers and Operations
© Mometrix Media – flashcardsecrets.com/teas
ATI TEAS Mathematics

Solve the following inequality: $7x > 5$.

Let d stand for the sales from dairy products. Let v stand for the sales from vegetables. One third of the sales from dairy products is the expression $\frac{d}{3}$. One half of the sales from vegetables is the expression $\frac{v}{2}$. The sum of these expressions should be greater than the monthly payment for the farm. An inequality for this is $\frac{d}{3} + \frac{v}{2} > P$.

To write out an **inequality**, you may need to translate a sentence into an inequality. This translation is putting the words into symbols. When translating, choose a variable to stand for the unknown value. Then, change the words or phrases into symbols.

For example, the sum of 2 and a number is at most 12.

So, you would write: $2 + b \leq 12$.

Let c stand for the number of CDs that Fred buys. Also, let D stand for the cost of each DVD that Fred buys. The expression $12c$ gives the cost of the CDs, and the expression $2D$ gives the cost of the DVDs. So the equation $12c + 2D = 60$ represents the situation described.

Even though you don't know the value for the time it took, you know it's the same for both players. When you have a quantity and a rate, dividing the quantity by the rate gives you the time. So divide each player's number of made shots by their rate and set those values equal. Luke made 20 shots at a rate of x shots per minute: $\frac{20}{x}$. John made 30 shots at a rate of $x + 5$ shots per minute (5 shots per minute more than Luke): $\frac{30}{x+5}$. Set these two values equal to one another because they both represent the amount of time it took to make the shots:
$$\frac{30}{x+5} = \frac{20}{x}$$
Cross multiply the proportion: $30x = 20(x + 5)$
Then, distribute the 20 across the parentheses: $30x = 20x + 100$
Now, you can subtract 20x from both sides of the equation, and you are left with: $10x = 100$
So, you can divide both sides by 10: $\frac{10x}{10} = \frac{100}{10}$
Now, you are left with: $x = 10$. So, Luke's speed was 10 shots per minute. Then, John's speed was 15 shots per minute.

To solve for x, divide both sides by 7, and the solution is $x > \frac{5}{7}$.

Solving inequalities can be done with the same rules as for solving equations. However, when multiplying or dividing by a negative number, the direction of the **inequality sign** must be flipped or **reversed**.

Solve $10 > -2x + 4$.

Graph the solution to the inequality: $10 > -2x + 4$.

How can the following be simplified?
$$\frac{\frac{2}{5}}{\frac{4}{7}}$$

How can the following be simplified?
$$\frac{1}{4} + \frac{3}{6}$$

How can the following be simplified?
$$\frac{7}{8} - \frac{8}{16}$$

How can the following be simplified?
$$\frac{1}{2} + \left(3\left(\frac{3}{4}\right) - 2\right) + 4$$

To graph an inequality, you make a **number line**. Then, put a circle around the value that is being compared to x. If you are graphing a *greater than* or *less than* inequality, the circle remains open. This stands for all of the values except -3. If the inequality is *greater than or equal to* or *less than or equal to*, you draw a closed circle around the value. This would stand for all of the values including the number.

Finally, look over the values that the solution stands for. Then, shade the number line in the needed direction. This example calls for graphing all of the values greater than -3. This is all of the numbers to the right of -3. So, you shade this area on the number line.

The opposite of addition is subtraction. So, subtract 4 from both sides. This gives you $6 > -2x$. Next, the opposite of multiplication is division. So, divide both sides by -2. Don't forget to flip the inequality symbol because you are dividing by a negative number. Now, you have $-3 < x$. You can rewrite this as $x > -3$.

Fractions with common denominators can be easily added or subtracted. Recall that the denominator is the bottom number in the fraction and that the numerator is the top number in the fraction.

The denominators of $\frac{1}{4}$ and $\frac{3}{6}$ are 4 and 6, respectively. The lowest common denominator of 4 and 6 is 12 because 12 is the least common multiple of 4 (multiples 4, 8, 12, 16, …) and 6 (multiples 6, 12, 18, 24, …). Convert each fraction to its equivalent with the newly found common denominator of 12.

$\frac{1 \times 3}{4 \times 3} = \frac{3}{12}; \frac{3 \times 2}{6 \times 2} = \frac{6}{12}$.

Now that the fractions have the same denominator, you can add them.

$\frac{3}{12} + \frac{6}{12} = \frac{9}{12}$.

Be sure to write your answer in lowest terms. Both 9 and 12 can be divided by 3, so the answer is $\frac{3}{4}$.

Dividing a fraction by a fraction may appear tricky, but it's not if you write out your steps carefully. Follow these steps to divide a fraction by a fraction.

Step 1: Rewrite the problem as a multiplication problem. Dividing by a fraction is the same as multiplying by its **reciprocal**, also known as its **multiplicative inverse**. The product of a number and its reciprocal is 1. Because $\frac{4}{7}$ times $\frac{7}{4}$ is 1, these numbers are reciprocals. Note that reciprocals can be found by simply interchanging the numerators and denominators. So, rewriting the problem as a multiplication problem gives $\frac{2}{5} \times \frac{7}{4}$.

Step 2: Perform multiplication of the fractions by multiplying the numerators by each other and the denominators by each other. In other words, multiply across the top and then multiply across the bottom.

$$\frac{2}{5} \times \frac{7}{4} = \frac{2 \times 7}{5 \times 4} = \frac{14}{20}$$

Step 3: Make sure the fraction is reduced to lowest terms. Both 14 and 20 can be divided by 2.

$$\frac{14}{20} = \frac{14 \div 2}{20 \div 2} = \frac{7}{10}$$

The answer is $\frac{7}{10}$.

When simplifying expressions, first perform operations within groups. Within the set of parentheses are multiplication and subtraction operations. Perform the multiplication first to get $\frac{1}{2} + \left(\frac{9}{4} - 2\right) + 4$.

Then, subtract two to obtain $\frac{1}{2} + \frac{1}{4} + 4$. Finally, perform addition from left to right: $\frac{1}{2} + \frac{1}{4} + 4 = \frac{2}{4} + \frac{1}{4} + \frac{16}{4} = \frac{19}{4}$.

Fractions with common denominators can be easily added or subtracted. Recall that the denominator is the bottom number in the fraction and that the numerator is the top number in the fraction.

The denominators of $\frac{7}{8}$ and $\frac{8}{16}$ are 8 and 16, respectively. The lowest common denominator of 8 and 16 is 16 because 16 is the least common multiple of 8 (multiples 8, 16, 24 …) and 16 (multiples 16, 32, 48, …). Convert each fraction to its equivalent with the newly found common denominator of 16.

$$\frac{7 \times 2}{8 \times 2} = \frac{14}{16} \qquad \frac{8 \times 1}{16 \times 1} = \frac{8}{16}$$

Now that the fractions have the same denominator, you can subtract them.

$$\frac{14}{16} - \frac{8}{16} = \frac{6}{16}$$

Be sure to write your answer in lowest terms. Both 6 and 16 can be divided by 2, so the answer is $\frac{3}{8}$.

Numbers and Operations
© Mometrix Media – flashcardsecrets.com/teas
ATI TEAS Mathematics

How can the following simplified?

$$0.22 + 0.5 - (5.5 + 3.3 \div 3)$$

Numbers and Operations
© Mometrix Media – flashcardsecrets.com/teas
ATI TEAS Mathematics

How can the following be simplified?

$$\frac{3}{2} + (4(0.5) - 0.75) + 2$$

Numbers and Operations
© Mometrix Media – flashcardsecrets.com/teas
ATI TEAS Mathematics

How can the following be simplified?

$$1.45 + 1.5 + (6 - 9 \div 2) + 45$$

Data Interpretation
© Mometrix Media – flashcardsecrets.com/teas
ATI TEAS Mathematics

What is statistics?

Data Interpretation
© Mometrix Media – flashcardsecrets.com/teas
ATI TEAS Mathematics

Define *data*, *quantitative data*, and *qualitative data*.

Data Interpretation
© Mometrix Media – flashcardsecrets.com/teas
ATI TEAS Mathematics

What is the difference between discrete data and continuous data?

First, simplify within the parentheses:
$\frac{3}{2} + (2 - 0.75) + 2 =$

$$\frac{3}{2} + 1.25 + 2$$

Finally, change the fraction to a decimal and perform addition from left to right:
$$1.5 + 1.25 + 2 = 4.75$$

First, evaluate the terms in the parentheses (5.5 + 3.3 ÷ 3) using order of operations. $3.3 \div 3 = 1.1$, and $5.5 + 1.1 = 6.6$.

Next, rewrite the problem: $0.22 + 0.5 - 6.6$.

Finally, add and subtract from left to right: $0.22 + 0.5 = 0.72$; $0.72 - 6.6 = -5.88$. The answer is -5.88.

Statistics is the branch of mathematics that deals with collecting, recording, interpreting, illustrating, and analyzing large amounts of **data**.

First, evaluate the terms in the parentheses using proper order of operations.
$$1.45 + 1.5 + (6 - 4.5) + 45$$
$$1.45 + 1.5 + 1.5 + 45$$

Finally, add from left to right.
$$1.45 + 1.5 + 1.5 + 45 = 49.45$$

Discrete data – information that can be expressed only by a specific value, such as whole or half numbers; For example, since people can be counted only in whole numbers, a population count would be discrete data.

Continuous data – information (such as time and temperature) that can be expressed by any value within a given range

Data – the collective name for pieces of information (singular is datum).

Quantitative data – measurements (such as length, mass, and speed) that provide information about quantities in numbers

Qualitative data – information (such as colors, scents, tastes, and shapes) that cannot be measured using numbers

Data Interpretation

What is the difference between primary data and secondary data?

Data Interpretation

What is the difference between ordinal data and nominal data?

Data Interpretation

What is a bar graph?

Data Interpretation

What is a line graph?

Data Interpretation

What is a pictograph?

Data Interpretation

What is a pie chart?

Ordinal data – information that can be placed in numerical order, such as age or weight

Nominal data – information that cannot be placed in numerical order, such as names or places.

Primary data – information that has been collected directly from a survey, investigation, or experiment, such as a questionnaire or the recording of daily temperatures; Primary data that has not yet been organized or analyzed is called raw data.

Secondary data – information that has been collected, sorted, and processed by the researcher

A **line graph** is a graph that connects points to show how data increases or decreases over time. The time line is the **horizontal axis**. The connecting lines between data points on the graph are a way to more clearly show how the data changes.

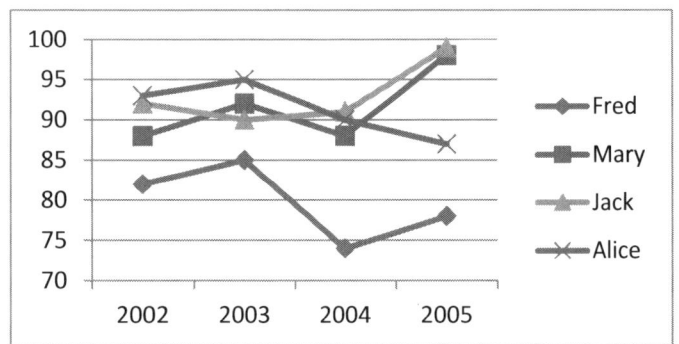

A **bar graph** is a graph that uses bars to compare data, as if each bar were a ruler being used to measure the data. The graph includes a **scale** that identifies the units being measured.

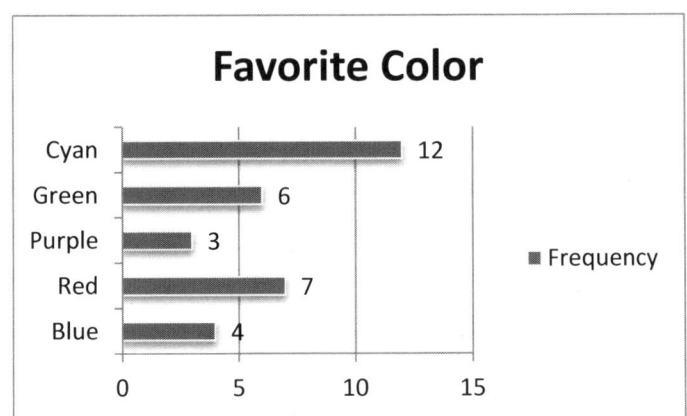

A **pie chart** or circle graph is a diagram used to compare parts of a whole.

A **pictograph** is a graph that uses pictures or symbols to show data. The pictograph will have a **key** to identify what each symbol represents.

Generally, each symbol stands for one or more objects.

Data Interpretation

How is a pie chart divided?

Data Interpretation

A group of students were surveyed on their favorite colors. The percentages were 38% for Cyan, 22% for Red, 19% for Purple, 13% for Blue, and 9% for Green. How would a pie chart represent this information?

Data Interpretation

Explain the features, and function of a histogram.

Data Interpretation

What is a stem and leaf plot?

Data Interpretation

What is an advantage of a stem and leaf plot over a histogram when reviewing a subset of numbers (e.g., 10s, 20s, 30s)?

Data Interpretation

Use all of the test scores from the line graph example to put together a stem and leaf plot.
(Test Scores in 70s: 74 and 78)
(Scores in 80s: 82, 85, 87, 88, and 88)
(Scores in 90s: 90, 90, 91, 92, 92, 93, 95, 98, and 99)

A pie chart representing this information would look something like this:

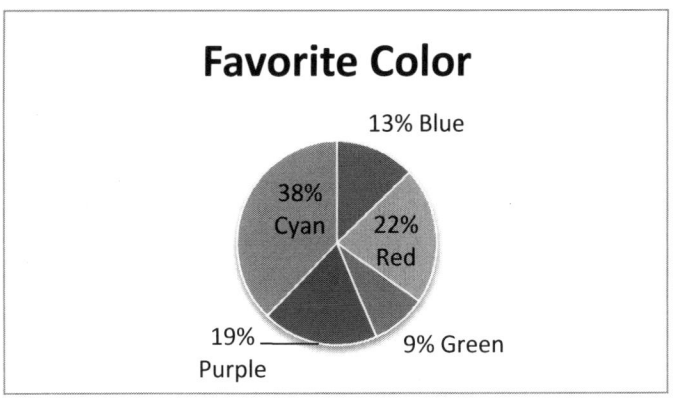

The full pie represents the whole, and it is divided into sectors where each represents something that is a part of the whole.

Each sector or slice of the pie is either labeled to indicate what it represents, or explained on a key associated with the chart. The size of each slice is determined by the *percentage of the whole* that the associated quantity represents.

Numerically, the angle measurement of each sector can be computed by solving the proportion: $x/360 =$ part/whole.

A **stem-and-leaf plot** can outline groups of data that fall into a range of values.

Each piece of data is split into two parts: the first, or left, part is called the stem. The second, or right, part is called the leaf. Each **stem** is listed in a column from smallest to largest.

Each **leaf** that has the common stem is listed in that stem's row from smallest to largest.

For example, in a set of two-digit numbers, the digit in the tens place is the stem. So, the digit in the ones place is the leaf.

A **histogram** is a special type of bar graph where the data are grouped in **intervals** (for example 20–29, 30–39, 40–49, etc.). The **frequency**, or number of times a value occurs in each interval, is indicated by the height of the bar. The intervals do not have to be the same amount but usually are (all data in ranges of 10 or all in ranges of 5, for example). The smaller the intervals, the more detailed the information.

4.5		
4.1		
4.0		
4.9	5.0	
4.6	5.1	
4.3	5.6	
4.8	5.9	

Using all of the test scores from the line graph, we can put together a stem and leaf plot:

Test Scores								
7	4	8						
8	2	5	7	8	8			
9	0	0	1	2	2	3	5	8	9

In this example, you can see that almost half of the students scored in the 80s. Also, all of the data has been maintained. These plots can be used for larger numbers as well. However, they work better for *small sets of data*.

With a stem and leaf plot, you can see which subset of numbers (10s, 20s, 30s, etc.) is the largest.

This information can be found by looking at a histogram. However, a stem and leaf plot also lets you look closer and see which values fall in that range.

Data Interpretation

© Mometrix Media – flashcardsecrets.com/teas
ATI TEAS Mathematics

How are scatter plots useful?

Data Interpretation

© Mometrix Media – flashcardsecrets.com/teas
ATI TEAS Mathematics

What are regressions and simple regressions?

Data Interpretation

© Mometrix Media – flashcardsecrets.com/teas
ATI TEAS Mathematics

How are positive linear and negative linear scatter plots drawn?

Data Interpretation

© Mometrix Media – flashcardsecrets.com/teas
ATI TEAS Mathematics

How are nonlinear exponential and nonlinear quadratic scatter plots drawn?

Data Interpretation

© Mometrix Media – flashcardsecrets.com/teas
ATI TEAS Mathematics

Use this graph to determine the range of the age of the patients.

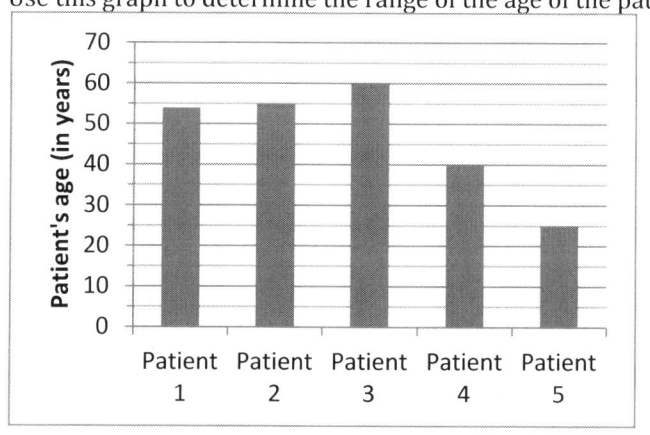

Data Interpretation

© Mometrix Media – flashcardsecrets.com/teas
ATI TEAS Mathematics

The patient's minimum measured heart rate occurred at what time? The patient's maximum measured heart rate occurred at what time? At what times during the day did the patient have the same measured heart rate? What trends, if any, can you find about the patient's heart rate throughout the day?

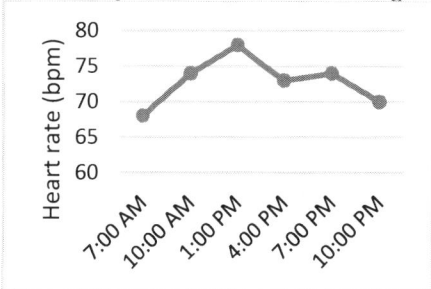

A **simple regression** is a regression that uses an independent variable.

A **regression** is a chart that is used to predict future events. Linear scatter plots may be positive or negative. Many nonlinear scatter plots are exponential or quadratic.

Scatter plots are useful for knowing the types of functions that are given with the data. Also, they are helpful for finding the simple regression.

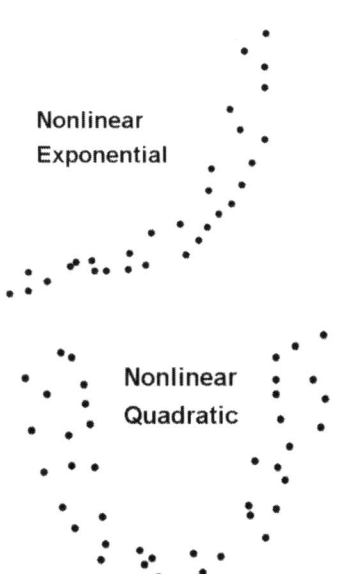

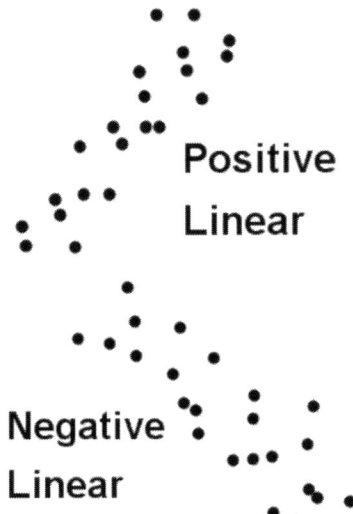

The patient's minimum measured heart rate occurred at the lowest data point on the graph, which is 68 bpm at 7:00 AM.

The patient's maximum measured heart rate occurred at the highest data point on the graph, which is 78 bpm at 1:00 PM.

The patient had the same measured heart rate of 74 bpm at 10:00 AM and 7:00 PM.

The patient's heart rate increased through the morning to early afternoon, and generally declined as the afternoon progressed.

Use the graph to find the age of each patient:
Patient 1 is 54 years old
Patient 2 is 55 years old
Patient 3 is 60 years old
Patient 4 is 40 years old
and Patient 5 is 25 years old.

The age range is the age of the oldest patient minus the age of the youngest patient. In other words, 60 – 25 = 35. The age range is 35 years.

Data Interpretation

In a drug study containing 100 patients, a new cholesterol drug was found to decrease low-density lipoprotein (LDL) levels in 25% of the patients. In a second study containing 50 patients, the same drug administered at the same dosage was found to decrease LDL levels in 50% of the patients.

Are the results of these two studies **consistent** with one another?

Data Interpretation

A nurse found the heart rates of eleven different patients to be 76, 80, 90, 86, 70, 76, 72, 88, 88, 68, and 88 beats per minute. Organize this information in a table.

Data Interpretation

What are variables?

Data Interpretation

What is the difference between independent variables and dependent variables?

Data Interpretation

Identify the independent variable and the dependent variable in the following question: If Ray earns $10 an hour, how much would he earn working 36 hours?

Data Interpretation

Solve the following question: If Ray earns $10 an hour, how much he would earn working 36 hours?

There are several ways to organize data in a table. The table below is an example.

Patient Number	Heart Rate (bpm)
1	76
2	80
3	90
4	86
5	70
6	76
7	72
8	88
9	88
10	68
11	88

When making a table, be sure to label the columns and rows appropriately.

Even though in both studies 25 people (25% of 100 is 25 and 50% of 50 is 25) showed improvements in their LDL levels, the results of the studies are inconsistent.

The results of the second study indicate that the drug has a much higher efficacy (desired result) than the results of the first study. Because 50 out of 150 total patients showed improvement on the medication, one could argue that the drug is effective in one third (or approximately 33%) of patients. However, one should be wary of the reliability of results when they're not **reproducible** from one study to the next and when the **sample size** is fairly low.

An **independent variable** is an input into a system that may take on values freely. **Dependent variables** are those that change as a consequence of changes in other values in the equation.

A **variable** is a symbol, usually an alphabetic character, designating a *value that may change* within the scope of a given problem. Variables can be described as either independent or dependent variables.

Once you have the equation for the function, you can choose any number of hours to find the corresponding amount that he earns.

If you want to know how much he would earn working 36 hours, you would substitute 36 in for x and multiply to find that he would earn $360.

This can be represented by the expression $10x$, where x is equal to the number of hours that Ray works. The value of x represents the number of hours because it is the independent variable, or the amount that you can choose and can manipulate.

To find out how much money y, he earns in x hours, you would write the equation, $10x = y$. The variable y is the dependent variable because it depends on x and cannot be manipulated.

A patient told a doctor she feels fine after running one mile but that her knee starts hurting after running two miles. Her knee throbs after running three miles and swells after running four.

Identify the independent and dependent variables with regard to the distance she runs and her level of pain.

What is bivariate data?

What can the variables tell you in bivariate data?

What is the mean or arithmetic average of a data set?

When is the mean most useful?

Identify if the mean the best way to solve the following or name an alternative:
The data set (1, 3, 6, 8, 100, 800), the mean is $\frac{1+3+6+8+100+800}{6} = 153$.

Bivariate data is data *from two different variables*. The prefix *bi-* means *two*. In a **scatter plot**, each value in the set of data is put on a grid. This is similar to the Cartesian plane where each axis represents one of the two variables.

An independent variable is one that does not depend on any other variables in the situation. In this case, the distance the patient runs would be considered the independent variable. The dependent variable would be her level of pain because it depends on how far she runs.

The **mean** is the *average of the data points*; that is, it is the sum of the data points divided by the number of data points. Mathematically, the mean of a set of data points $\{x_1, x_2, x_3, \ldots x_n\}$ can be written as $\bar{X} = \sum \frac{X}{N}$.

For instance, for the data set (1, 3, 6, 8, 100, 800), the mean is $\frac{1+3+6+8+100+800}{6} = 153$.

When you look at the pattern made by the points on the grid, you may know if there is a relationship between the two variables. Also, you may know what that relationship is and if it exists.

The variables may be directly proportionate, inversely proportionate, or show no proportion. Also, you may be able to see if the data is linear. If the data is linear, you can find an equation to show the two variables.

In this example, the data shows much **variation**.

Thus, the mean is not the best measure of central tendency to use, when interpreting the data.

With this data set, the **median** will give a more complete picture of the distribution.

The mean is most useful, when data is approximately normal and does not include extreme **outliers** (data values that are unusually high or unusually low compared to the rest of the data values).

Data Interpretation

What is the median of a data set?

Data Interpretation

What is the mode?

Data Interpretation

What can be done with a data set where there are multiple modes?

Data Interpretation

How is the mode of a data set useful?

Data Interpretation

What is the range of a data set?

Data Interpretation

What is symmetry in reference to data distribution?

The **mode** is the value that appears *most often in the data set*.

For instance, for the data set {2, 6, 4, 9, 4, 5, 7, 6, 4, 1, 5, 6, 7, 5, 6}, the mode is 6: the number 6 appears four times in the data set, while the next most frequent values, 4 and 5, appear only three times each.

The mode is useful to get a general sense of the *shape of the distribution*; it shows where the peaks of the distribution are. More information is necessary to get a more detailed description of the full shape.

Symmetry is a characteristic of the shape of the plotted data. Specifically, it refers to how well the data on one side of the median **mirrors** the data on the other side.

The **median** is the value *in the middle of the data set*, in the sense that 50% of the data points lie above the median and 50% of the data points lie below. The median can be determined by simply putting the data points in order, and selecting the data point in the middle. If there is an even number of data points, then the median is the average of the middle two data points.

For instance, for the data set {1, 3, 6, 8, 100, 800}, the median is $\frac{6+8}{2} = 7$.

It is possible for a data set to have more than one mode: in the data set {11, 14, 17, 16, 11, 17, 12, 14, 17, 14, 13}, 14 and 17 are both modes, appearing three times each.

In the extreme case of a uniform distribution—a distribution in which all values appear with equal probability—all values in the data set are modes.

The range of a distribution is the *difference between the highest and lowest values in the distribution*.

For example, in the data set (1, 3, 5, 7, 9, 11), the highest and lowest values are 11 and 1, respectively. The range then would be calculated as 11 − 1 = 10.

Data Interpretation

What is skewed data?

Data Interpretation

What is left skewed data and right skewed data?

Data Interpretation

How can the names "left skewness" and "right skewness" seem counterintuitive?

Data Interpretation

Which data distribution is skewed right and which is skewed left?

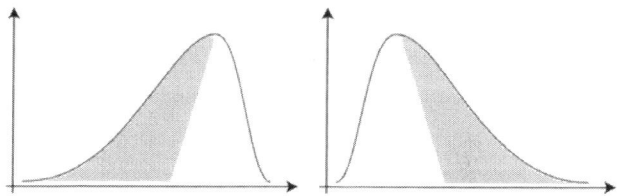

Data Interpretation

What is the difference between unimodal and bimodal distribution?

Data Interpretation

What is a uniform distribution?

A data set that is *skewed left* has more of its values to the left of the peak, while a set that is *skewed right* has more of its values to the right of the peak.

A **skewed** data set is one that has a distinctly longer or fatter tail on one side of the peak or the other.

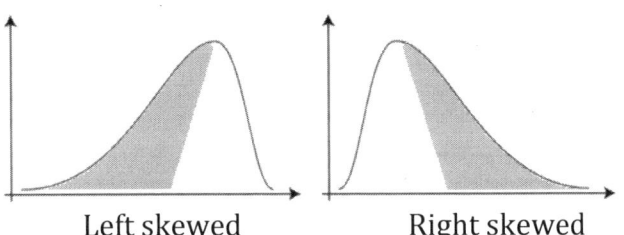
Left skewed   Right skewed

When actually looking at the graph, these names may seem counterintuitive since, in a left-skewed data set, the bulk of the values seem to be on the right side of the graph, and vice versa.

However, if the graph is viewed strictly in relation to the peak, the direction of skewness makes more sense.

A uniform distribution is a distribution in which there is *no distinct peak or variation in the data*. No values or ranges are particularly more common than any other values or ranges.

If a distribution has a single peak, it would be considered **unimodal**. If it has two discernible peaks it would be considered **bimodal**.

Bimodal distributions may be an indication that the set of data being considered is actually the combination of two sets of data with significant differences.

What is a quadrilateral?

What is a parallelogram?

What is a trapezoid?

What is a rectangle?

What is a rhombus?

What is a square?

Parallelogram: A quadrilateral that has exactly two pairs of opposite **parallel** sides. The sides that are parallel are also **congruent**. The opposite interior angles are always congruent, and the consecutive interior angles are **supplementary**. The **diagonals** of a parallelogram bisect each other. Each diagonal divides the parallelogram into two congruent triangles.

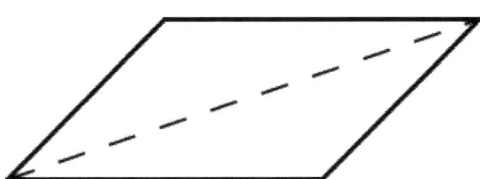

Quadrilateral: A closed two-dimensional geometric figure composed of exactly four straight sides. The sum of the interior angles of any quadrilateral is 360°.

Rectangle: A parallelogram with four right angles. All rectangles are parallelograms, but not all parallelograms are rectangles. The diagonals of a rectangle are congruent.

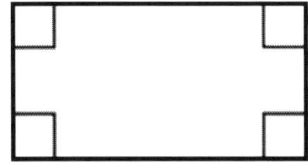

Trapezoid: Traditionally, a quadrilateral that has exactly one pair of parallel sides. Some math texts define trapezoid as a quadrilateral that has at least one pair of parallel sides. Because there are no rules governing the second pair of sides, there are no rules that apply to the properties of the diagonals of a trapezoid.

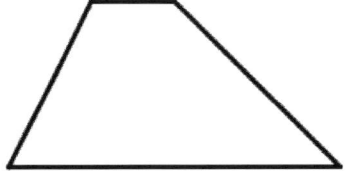

Square: A parallelogram with four right angles and four congruent sides. All squares are also parallelograms, rhombuses, and rectangles. The diagonals of a square are congruent and perpendicular to each other.

Rhombus: A parallelogram with four congruent sides. All rhombuses are parallelograms, but not all parallelograms are rhombuses. The diagonals of a rhombus are **perpendicular** to each other.

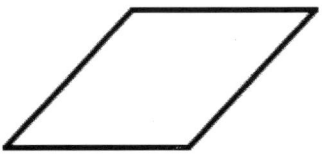

Measurement

How can a quadrilateral also be a parallelogram?

Measurement

How can a quadrilateral also be a rhombus?

Measurement

How can a parallelogram also be a rectangle?

Measurement

How can a rhombus also be a square?

Measurement

Explain the center of a circle and the radius of a circle.

Measurement

Explain the diameter of a circle.

A quadrilateral whose diagonals are perpendicular bisectors of each other is a **rhombus**. A quadrilateral whose opposite sides (both pairs) are parallel and congruent is a rhombus.

A quadrilateral whose diagonals bisect each other is a **parallelogram**. A quadrilateral whose opposite sides are parallel (2 pairs of parallel sides) is a parallelogram.

A rhombus with one right angle is a **square**.

Because the rhombus is a special form of a parallelogram, the rules about the angles of a parallelogram also apply to the rhombus.

A parallelogram that has a right angle is a **rectangle**.

(Consecutive angles of a parallelogram are supplementary. Therefore if there is one right angle in a parallelogram, there are four right angles in that parallelogram.)

The **diameter** is a line segment that passes through the center of the circle and has both endpoints on the circle. The length of the diameter is exactly twice the length of the radius. (Segment XZ in the diagram below.)

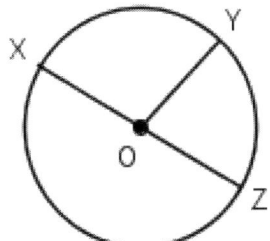

The **center** is the single point inside the circle that is **equidistant** from every point on the circle. (Point O in the diagram below.)

The **radius** is a line segment that joins the center of the circle and any one point on the circle. All radii of a circle are equal. (Segments OX, OY, and OZ in the diagram below.)

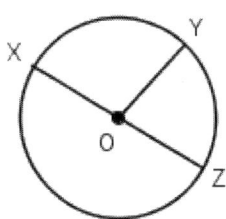

Measurement

Explain an arc of a circle, and explain how a sector in a circle is formed.

Measurement

What are central angles and minor arcs?

Measurement

What are major arcs and semicircles?

Measurement

What are chords and secants?

Measurement

What are inscribed angles and intercepted arcs?

Measurement

What is the relationship between the measure of an intercepted arc and the measure of an inscribed angle?

A **central angle** is an angle whose **vertex** is the center of a circle and whose legs intercept an arc of the circle. Angle *XOY* in the diagram below is a central angle. A **minor arc** is an arc that has a measure less than 180°. The measure of a central angle is equal to the measure of the minor arc it intercepts.

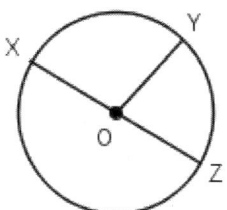

An **arc** is a portion of a circle. Specifically, an arc is the set of points between and including two points on a circle. An arc does not contain any points inside the circle.

When a segment is drawn from the endpoints of an arc to the center of the circle, a **sector** is formed.

A **chord** is a line segment that has both endpoints on a circle. In the diagram below, $\overline{EB}$ is a chord.

Secant: A line that passes through a circle and contains a chord of that circle. In the diagram below, $\overleftrightarrow{EB}$ is a secant and contains chord $\overline{EB}$.

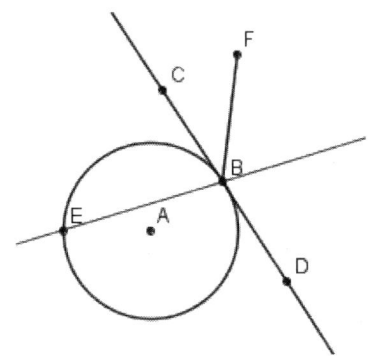

A **major arc** is an arc having a measure of at least 180°. The measure of the major arc can be found by subtracting the measure of the central angle from 360°.

A **semicircle** is an arc whose endpoints are the endpoints of the diameter of a circle. A semicircle is exactly half of a circle.

The measure of the intercepted arc is exactly twice the measure of the inscribed angle. In the diagram below, angle *ABC* is an inscribed angle. $\widehat{AC} = 2(m\angle ABC)$.

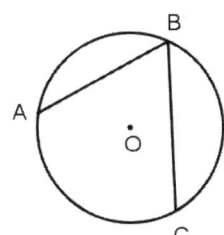

An **inscribed angle** is an angle whose vertex lies on a circle and whose legs contain chords of that circle.

The portion of the circle intercepted by the legs of the angle is called the **intercepted arc**.

What is arc length?

What is the formula for arc length?

What is the difference between a sector and the arc length of a circle?

How can the area of a sector of a circle be found?

How can the area of a sector of a circle be found when the central angle is in degrees?

What can be done to find the *perimeter* and the *area* of any triangle?

The formula for arc length is $s = \frac{\pi r \theta}{180°}$ where s is the arc length, r is the length of the radius, and θ is the angular measure of the arc in degrees, or $s = r\theta$, where θ is the angular measure of the arc in radians (2π radians $= 360$ degrees).

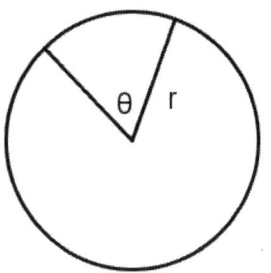

The **arc length** is the length of that portion of the circumference between two points on the circle.

The **area** of a sector of a circle is found by the formula $A = \frac{\theta r^2}{2}$, where A is the area, θ is the measure of the central angle in radians, and r is the radius.

A **sector** is the portion of a circle formed by two radii and their intercepted arc.

While the arc length is exclusively the points that are also on the circumference of the circle, the sector is the entire area bounded by the arc and the two radii.

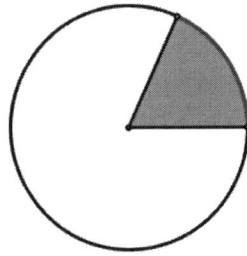

The **perimeter** of any triangle is found by summing the three side lengths; $P = a + b + c$. For an **equilateral triangle**, this is the same as $P = 3s$, where s is any side length, since all three sides are the same length.

The **area** of any triangle can be found by taking half the product of one side length (base or b) and the perpendicular distance from that side to the opposite vertex (height or h). In equation form, $A = \frac{1}{2}bh$.

To find the area when the central angle is in degrees, use the formula, $= \frac{\theta \pi r^2}{360}$, where θ is the measure of the central angle in degrees and r is the radius.

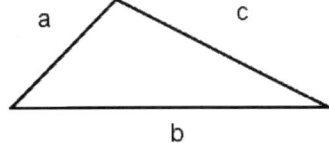

Measurement
ATI TEAS Mathematics

What can be done to find the *perimeter* and the *area* of a square?

Measurement
ATI TEAS Mathematics

What is the fastest way to find the perimeter of a square?

Measurement
ATI TEAS Mathematics

What can be done to find the *perimeter* and the *area* of a rectangle?

Measurement
ATI TEAS Mathematics

What can be done to find the *perimeter* and the *area* of a parallelogram?

Measurement
ATI TEAS Mathematics

How can you find the *perimeter* and the *area* of a trapezoid?

Measurement
ATI TEAS Mathematics

How can you find the *perimeter* and the *area* of a circle?

Because all four sides are equal in a square, it is faster to multiply the length of one side by 4 than to add the same number four times. You could use the formulas for rectangles and get the same answer.

The **perimeter** of a square is found by using the formula $P = 4s$, where s is the length of one side.

The **area** of a square is found by using the formula $A = s^2$, where and s is the length of one side.

The **perimeter** of a parallelogram is found by the formula $P = 2a + 2b$ or $P = 2(a + b)$, where a and b are the lengths of the two sides.

The **area** of a parallelogram is found by the formula $A = bh$, where b is the length of the base, and h is the height.

Note that the base and height correspond to the length and width in a rectangle, so this formula would apply to rectangles as well.

Do not confuse the height of a parallelogram with the length of the second side. The two are only the same measure in the case of a rectangle.

The **perimeter** of a rectangle is found by the formula $P = 2l + 2w$ or $P = 2(l + w)$, where l is the length, and w is the width.

It may be easier to add the length and width first and then double the result, as in the second formula.

The **area** of a rectangle is found by the formula $A = lw$, where A is the area of the rectangle, l is the length (usually considered to be the longer side) and w is the width (usually considered to be the shorter side). The numbers for l and w are interchangeable.

The **perimeter** (**circumference**) of a circle is found by the formula $C = 2\pi r$, where r is the radius. Again, remember to convert the diameter if you are given that measure rather than the radius.

The **area** of a circle is found by the formula $A = \pi r^2$, where r is the length of the radius. If the diameter of the circle is given, remember to divide it in half to get the length of the radius before proceeding.

The **perimeter** of a trapezoid is found by the formula $P = a + b_1 + c + b_2$, where a, b_1, c, and b_2 are the four sides of the trapezoid.

The **area** of a trapezoid is found by the formula $A = \frac{1}{2}h(b_1 + b_2)$, where h is the height (segment joining and perpendicular to the parallel bases), and b_1 and b_2 are the two parallel sides (bases). Do not use one of the other two sides as the height unless that side is also perpendicular to the parallel bases.

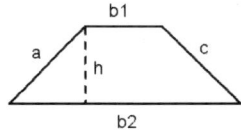

Measurement

What is the formula for finding the *surface area* and the *volume* of any prism?

Measurement

What is the formula for finding the *surface area* and the *volume* of a sphere?

Measurement

Dwight has a beach ball with a radius of 9 inches. He is planning to wrap the ball with wrapping paper.
How many square feet of wrapping paper are needed to cover the surface of the ball?

Measurement

What is the formula for finding the *surface area* and the *volume* of a cube?

Measurement

What is the formula for finding the *surface area* and the *volume* of a rectangular prism?

Measurement

What is the formula for finding the *surface area* and the *volume* of a cylinder?

The **surface area** of a sphere can be found by the formula $A = 4\pi r^2$, where r is the radius.

The **volume** of a sphere can be found with the formula $V = \frac{4}{3}\pi r^3$, where r is the radius. Both quantities are generally given in terms of π.

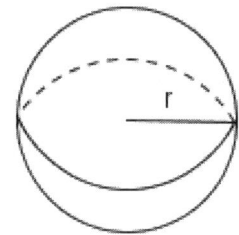

The **surface area** of any prism is the sum of the areas of both bases and all sides. It can be calculated as $SA = 2B + Ph$, where P is the perimeter of the base.

The **volume** of any prism is found with the formula $V = Bh$, where B is the area of the base, and h is the height. The perpendicular distance between the bases is the height.

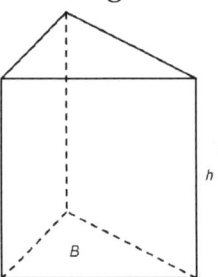

The **surface area** of a cube is calculated as $SA = 6s^2$, where SA is the total surface area and s is the length of a side.

The **volume** of a cube can be found with the formula $V = s^3$, where s is the length of a side.

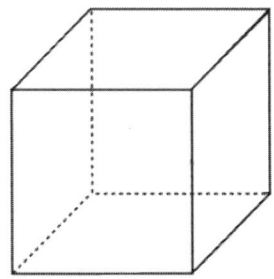

The surface area of a sphere may be calculated using the formula $SA = 4\pi r^2$. Substituting 9 for r gives $SA = 4\pi(9)^2$, which simplifies to $SA \approx 1017.36$. So the surface area of the ball is approximately 1017.36 square inches. There are twelve inches in a foot. So, there are $12^2 = 144$ square inches in a square foot.

To convert this measurement to square feet, the following proportion may be written and solved for x: $\frac{1}{144} = \frac{x}{1017.36}$. So $x \approx 7.07$, meaning it will take approximately 7.07 square feet of wrapping paper to cover the surface of the ball.

The **surface area** of a cylinder can be found by the formula $SA = 2\pi r^2 + 2\pi rh$. The first term is the base area multiplied by two, and the second term is the perimeter of the base multiplied by the height.

The **volume** of a cylinder can be found with the formula $V = \pi r^2 h$, where r is the radius, and h is the height.

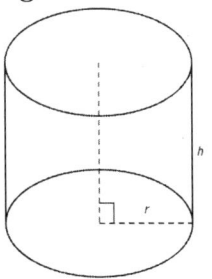

The **surface area** can be calculated as $SA = 2lw + 2hl + 2wh$ or $SA = 2(lw + hl + wh)$.

The **volume** of a rectangular prism can be found with the formula $V = lwh$, where V is the volume, l is the length, w is the width, and h is the height.

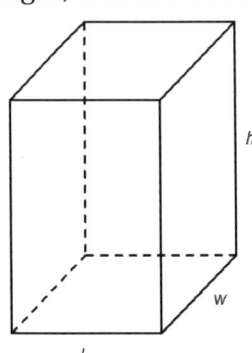

Measurement

What is the Cartesian Coordinate Plane?

Measurement

What are the attributes of the horizontal line and the vertical line on the coordinate plane?

Measurement

Draw a coordinate plane, and label the plane with the four **quadrants**: I, II, III, and IV.

Measurement

Place the following points on the coordinate plane:
A. (−4, −2) | B. (−1, 3) | C. (2, 2) | D. (3, −1)

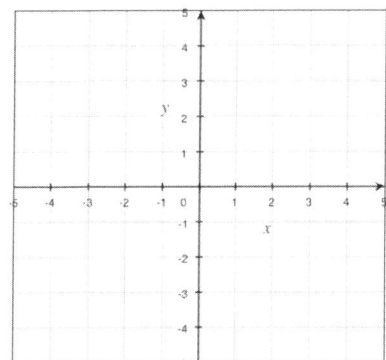

Measurement

The key on one map says that 2 inches on the map is 12 real miles. Find the distance of a route that is 5 inches long on the map.

Measurement

For measurement conversion, what needs to be done to go from a larger unit to a smaller unit and to go from a smaller unit to a larger unit?

The horizontal number line is known as the **x-axis**, with positive values to the right of the **origin**, and negative values to the left of the origin.

The vertical number line is known as the **y-axis**, with positive values above the origin, and negative values below the origin. Any point on the plane can be identified by an ordered pair in the form (x,y), called coordinates.

The x-value of the coordinate is called the **abscissa**, and the y-value of the coordinate is called the **ordinate**.

When algebraic functions and equations are shown graphically, they are usually shown on a *Cartesian Coordinate Plane*. The Cartesian coordinate plane consists of two number lines placed perpendicular to each other, and intersecting at the zero point, also known as the origin.

Answer

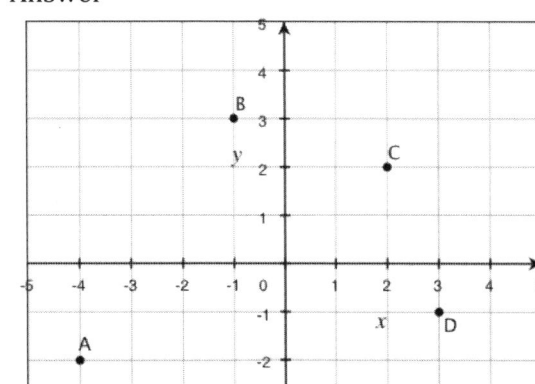

When going from a larger unit to a smaller unit, multiply the number of the known amount by the **equivalent amount**.

When going from a smaller unit to a larger unit, divide the number of the known amount by the equivalent amount.

A **proportion** is needed to show the map measurements and real distances. First, write a ratio that has the information in the key. The map measurement can be in the numerator, and the real distance can be in the denominator.

$$\frac{2 \text{ inches}}{12 \text{ miles}}$$

Next, write a ratio with the known map distance and the unknown real distance. The unknown number for miles can be represented with the letter m.

$$\frac{5 \text{ inches}}{m \text{ miles}}$$

Then, write out the ratios in a proportion and solve it for m.

$$\frac{2 \text{ inches}}{12 \text{ miles}} = \frac{5 \text{ inches}}{m \text{ miles}}$$

Now, you have $2m = 60$. So, you are left with $m = 30$. Thus, the route is 30 miles long.

Measurement

For measurement conversion, what are conversion fractions?

Measurement

Fill in the blanks:

1000 ___ (microgram)	___ mg
1000 mg (milligram)	1 __
1000 __ (_____)	1 kg

Measurement

Fill in the blanks:

1000 kg (kilogram)	1 _____
1000 __ (_____)	1 L
1000 um (micrometer)	1 ___

Measurement

Fill in the blanks:

____ mm (millimeter)	1 m
100 cm (centimeter)	1 __
1000 __ (_____)	1 km

Measurement

Fill in the blanks:

Unit	U.S. equivalent	Metric equivalent
	1 ____	2.54 centimeters
1 Foot	12 inches	__.____ meters
1 Yard	__ feet	0.914 meters
1 _____	5280 _____	1.609 kilometers

Measurement

Fill in the blanks:

Unit	U.S. equivalent	Metric equivalent
Ounce	8 drams	29.573 milliliters
Cup	8 _____	0.237 liter
____	16 ounces	__.____ liter
Quart	2 _____	0.946 liter
Gallon	__ quarts	3.785 liters

Measurement

1000 mcg (microgram)	1 mg
1000 mg (milligram)	1 g
1000 g (gram)	1 kg

In these fractions, one fraction is the **conversion factor**. The other fraction has the unknown amount in the numerator. So, the known value is placed in the denominator. Sometimes the second fraction has the known value from the problem in the numerator, and the unknown in the denominator.

Multiply the two fractions to get the converted measurement.

Measurement

1000 mm (millimeter)	1 m
100 cm (centimeter)	1 m
1000 m (meter)	1 km

Measurement

1000 kg (kilogram)	1 metric ton
1000 mL (milliliter)	1 L
1000 um (micrometer)	1 mm

Measurement

Unit	U.S. equivalent	Metric equivalent
Ounce	8 drams	29.573 milliliters
Cup	8 ounces	0.237 liter
Pint	16 ounces	0.473 liter
Quart	2 pints	0.946 liter
Gallon	4 quarts	3.785 liters

Measurement

Unit	U.S. equivalent	Metric equivalent
	1 inch	2.54 centimeters
1 Foot	12 inches	0.305 meters
1 Yard	3 feet	0.914 meters
1 Mile	5280 feet	1.609 kilometers

Measurement

Fill in the blanks:

Unit	U.S. equivalent	Metric equivalent
Ounce	___ drams	28.35 grams
_____	16 ounces	___.___ grams
Ton	2,000 _____	907.2 kilograms

Measurement

Fill in the blanks:

Unit	U.S. equivalent	Metric equivalent
1 tsp	1.333 fluid drams	5 milliliters
___ tsp	4 fluid drams	___ or ___ milliliters
2 ____	1 fluid ounce	30 milliliters
___ glass	8 fluid ounces	____ milliliters

Measurement

Measurement Conversion Practice Problems
a. Convert 1.4 meters to centimeters.
b. Convert 218 centimeters to meters.

Measurement

Measurement Conversion Practice Problems
a. Convert 42 inches to feet.
b. Convert 15 feet to yards.

Measurement

Measurement Conversion Practice Problems
a. How many pounds are in 15 kilograms?
b. How many pounds are in 80 ounces?

Measurement

Measurement Conversion Practice Problems
a. How many kilometers are in 2 miles?
b. How many centimeters are in 5 feet?

Measurement

Unit	U.S. equivalent	Metric equivalent
1 tsp	1.333 fluid drams	5 milliliters
3 tsp	4 fluid drams	15 or 16 milliliters
2 tbsp	1 fluid ounce	30 milliliters
1 glass	8 fluid ounces	240 milliliters

Measurement

Unit	U.S. equivalent	Metric equivalent
Ounce	16 drams	28.35 grams
Pound	16 ounces	453.6 grams
Ton	2,000 pounds	907.2 kilograms

a. $\frac{12 \text{ in}}{1 \text{ ft}} = \frac{42 \text{ in}}{x \text{ ft}}$. Cross multiply to get $12x = 42$, or $x = 3.5$. So, there are 42 inches in 3.5 feet.

a. $\frac{100 \text{ cm}}{1 \text{ m}} = \frac{x \text{ cm}}{1.4 \text{ m}}$. Cross multiply to get $x = 140$. So, there are 1.4 m in 140 cm.

b. $\frac{3 \text{ ft}}{1 \text{ yd}} = \frac{15 \text{ ft}}{x \text{ yd}}$. Cross multiply to get $3x = 15$, or $x = 5$. So, there are 15 feet in 5 yards.

b. $\frac{100 \text{ cm}}{1 \text{ m}} = \frac{218 \text{ cm}}{x \text{ m}}$. Cross multiply to get $100x = 218$, or $x = 2.18$. So, there are 218 cm in 2.18 m.

a. $2 \text{ miles} \times \frac{1.609 \text{ kilometers}}{1 \text{ mile}} = 3.218 \text{ kilometers}$

a. $15 \text{ kilograms} \times \frac{2.2 \text{ pounds}}{1 \text{ kilogram}} = 33 \text{ pounds}$

b. $5 \text{ feet} \times \frac{12 \text{ inches}}{1 \text{ foot}} \times \frac{2.54 \text{ centimeters}}{1 \text{ inch}} = 152.4 \text{ centimeters}$

b. $80 \text{ ounces} \times \frac{1 \text{ pound}}{16 \text{ ounces}} = 5 \text{ pounds}$

Measurement

Measurement Conversion Practice Problems
a. How many gallons are in 15.14 liters?
b. How many liters are in 8 quarts?

Measurement

Measurement Conversion Practice Problems
a. How many grams are in 13.2 pounds?
b. How many pints are in 9 gallons?

a. $13.2 \text{ pounds} \times \dfrac{1 \text{ kilogram}}{2.2 \text{ pounds}} \times \dfrac{1000 \text{ grams}}{1 \text{ kilogram}} =$ 6000 grams

b. $9 \text{ gallons} \times \dfrac{4 \text{ quarts}}{1 \text{ gallon}} \times \dfrac{2 \text{ pints}}{1 \text{ quarts}} = 72 \text{ pints}$

a. $15.14 \text{ liters} \times \dfrac{1 \text{ gallon}}{3.785 \text{ liters}} = 4 \text{ gallons}$

b. $8 \text{ quarts} \times \dfrac{1 \text{ gallon}}{4 \text{ quarts}} \times \dfrac{3.785 \text{ liters}}{1 \text{ gallon}} = 7.57 \text{ liters}$